Narrative ...

A Short-Term Treatment for
Traumatic Stress Disorders
2nd revised and expanded editon

Narrative Exposure Therapy

A Short-Term Treatment for Traumatic Stress Disorders

2nd revised and expanded edition

Maggie Schauer

Frank Neuner

Thomas Elbert

HOGREFE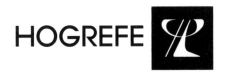

Library of Congress Cataloging in Publication
is available via the Library of Congress Marc Database under the
LC Control Number 2011927494

Library and Archives Canada Cataloguing in Publication

Schauer, Maggie
    Narrative exposure therapy : a short-term treatment for traumatic stress disorders / Maggie Schauer, Frank Neuner, Thomas Elbert.
-- 2nd rev. and expanded ed.

Includes bibliographical references.
ISBN 978-0-88937-388-4

    1. Post-traumatic stress disorder--Treatment. 2. Narrative therapy.
3. Victims of violent crimes--Rehabilitation. I. Neuner, Frank II. Elbert, Thomas III. Title.

RC552.P67S33 2011   616.85'210651   C2011-903035-7

PUBLISHING OFFICES
USA: Hogrefe Publishing, 875 Massachusetts Avenue, 7th Floor, Cambridge, MA 02139
              Phone (866) 823-4726, Fax (617) 354-6875, E-mail customerservice@hogrefe-publishing.com
EUROPE: Hogrefe Publishing, Rohnsweg 25, 37085 Göttingen, Germany
              Phone +49 551 49609-0, Fax +49 551 49609-88, E-mail publishing@hogrefe.com

SALES & DISTRIBUTION
USA: Hogrefe Publishing, Customer Services Department, 30 Amberwood Parkway, Ashland, OH 44805
              Phone (800) 228-3749, Fax (419) 281-6883, E-mail customerservice@hogrefe.com
EUROPE: Hogrefe Publishing, Rohnsweg 25, 37085 Göttingen, Germany
              Phone +49 551 49609-0, Fax +49 551 49609-88, E-mail publishing@hogrefe.com

OTHER OFFICES
CANADA: Hogrefe Publishing, 660 Eglinton Ave. East, Suite 119-514, Toronto, Ontario, M4G 2K2
SWITZERLAND: Hogrefe Publishing, Länggass-Strasse 76, CH-3000 Bern 9

Hogrefe Publishing
Incorporated and registered in the Commonwealth of Massachusetts, USA, and in Göttingen, Lower Saxony, Germany

Printed in Canada
ISBN 978-0-88937-388-4

Acknowledgments

This manual was written in cooperation with Dr. Elisabeth Schauer (vivo). We thank Drs. Brigitte Rockstroh, Claudia Catani, and Martina Ruf for helpful comments and continuous support of our work.

Research was supported by the European Refugee Fund, the Deutsche Forschungsgemeinschaft, and the nongovernmental organization vivo.

Cover Picture

The cover picture was taken by the therapist Dr. Claudia Catani (vivo) during a therapy session with a traumatized Sri Lankan child. The lifeline is a creative medium used in narrative exposure therapy (NET and KIDNET) that displays the chronological order of good (flowers) and bad or traumatic events (stones) in a survivor's biography (see Figure 12, "Lifeline of a Sudanese refugee woman," in Section 3.2.3).

Table of Contents

1 Introduction: Voices of Victims

Traumatized people become "stuck" in the horror they endured. Traumatic memories dominate the life of many survivors, who continue to live in fear and feel tormented, even when the threat is long gone. Their body and mind feel and act as if an ongoing threat endangers their survival. At the core of psychological trauma is the confusion of past and present. The intrusive memories of the traumatic events can create a world that seems more real than the actual reality. Survivors with traumatic stress disorders have never arrived in the present – have never reached the here and now. The result is the alienation of a wounded soul from life in the present and the future.

When severe pain and harm are purposefully inflicted by one human being on another, a breach of humanity has occurred. Even natural disasters and life-threatening accidents are sometimes viewed not as occasional occurrences that may happen to anyone but as deliberate and intentional acts of violence, and are therefore taken by the survivor to be a very personal attack.

Trauma destroys the human kernel that resides in moments or acts that occur within a social context: communication, speech, autobiographical remembrance, dignity, peace, and freedom. Trauma isolates the survivor, alienates life, and indeed freezes the flow of one's personal biography. In this introduction, we will listen to the voices of survivors of violent acts, of childhood abuse and neglect, and of torture, terror, and suffering:

> *A dream full of horror has not stopped visiting me, at sometimes frequent, sometimes longer, intervals: I am sitting in a peaceful relaxed environment, apparently without tension or affliction; yet I feel a deep and subtle anguish, the definite sensation of an impending threat. And, in fact, as the dream proceeds, slowly and brutally, each time in a different way, everything collapses and disintegrates around me, the scenery, the walls, the people, while the anguish becomes more intense and more precise. Now everything has changed into chaos; I am alone in the centre of a grey and turbid nothing, and now I know what this thing means, and I also know that I have always known it; I am in the Lager once more, and nothing is true outside the Lager. All the rest was a brief pause, a deception of the senses, a dream.... I have fallen into a rather serious depression. I ask you as a*

> *"proper doctor," what should I do? I feel the need for help but I do not know what sort.*
> Primo Levi, Auschwitz survivor, in a letter to his friend and doctor David Mendel, February 7, 1987 ("David Mendel", 2007; Gambetta, 1999; Levi, 1963)

Collective trauma remembrance must never be wiped out ('forgive, but don't forget'!), the horror can never be made undone and the autobiographic past can never be erased by psychotherapy, but the survivors' suffering can be reduced a great deal. Treatments that indeed lead to a reorganization of the fear network are of central importance: they can induce a long-term structural change in a patients memory and not only an inhibition of the fear network, with the constant threat of reactivation of the implicit fear network through trauma-associated triggers. The integration of traumatic events is especially important since trauma memories of a suffering individual can get reactivated throughout the lifespan. Stressors, similarities to the old event, that activate parts of the fear network that has been built by previous traumata lead to reactivation and as a consequence reactivation can lead to a relapse even after years without symptoms. As legend has it, Primo Levi told to Raabi Elio Toaff in a telephone conversation: "I can't go on with this life. My mother is ill with cancer and every time I look at her face I remember the faces of those men stretched on the benches at Auschwitz" (Gambetta, 1999).

Trauma subsists through the abnormal coding of memories. Conscious recollection of the past has become impossible, while barely noticeable traces sneak through attentional gates and evoke memories of the traumatic events so vivid and real that fear and horror have become routine. An "as-if" reenactment of the past becomes a piece of the present, a composite too terrible to utter aloud. Speechlessness from the terror results.

> *When I think of this time, fear is rising. In the past, we had to suppress it because of the permanent danger, but today I feel strange, because I only remember fragments. Why is that so? I feel as if a part of me is still hiding. I am staring into the darkness and only now and then something flashes up and lays open, a memory of my previous life.*
> Ervin Staub, child survivor of the Holocaust, in Stein (1993)

Continuous or complex trauma survivors have had to live through frequent interpersonal abuse often from early childhood on. It may take decades in these victims until the first distinct sensory intrusive memories surface, although they have had to endure a long life full of symptoms of "unknown" origin, of untold misery:

One day I looked in the mirror. On my arms and legs there was hardly any place where I had not cut or burned myself.... I was 30 years old. This time I was hospitalized for 14 weeks. It was my 57th stay as an inpatient in a psychiatric ward. I had suffered from eating disorders, bodily pains and drug abuse since 16 years by then. During the 2nd week, I suddenly experienced my first flashback of sexual abuse through my grandfather. I saw him raping me. After this stay, I had panic attacks and nightmares. More and more memories appeared. I realized that my father had done the same thing to me. I felt immense disgust. I slit my wrists; another attempt to die. After that, I stayed again for 5 months on a locked ward. Terrible fractions of memory of a time when I was sold to men in child-prostitution were haunting me. I wished I had succeeded to starve myself to death....
D. I., patient with borderline personality disorder, excerpt from a diagnostic interview at University of Konstanz' outpatient clinic, Center for Psychiatry Reichenau, Germany, 2010

The horror of the past – alive in the moment – can also take over the body and the mind. Listen to the voice of one woman describing those moments when the memories engulfed her being:

When I remember this body, so close to me, so ugly, so intimate, it is still as if there is a dark, bad, black thing entering me at the height of my stomach. It is a thing with arms, like an animal, like a snake, a winding being that enters me and turns around in me and twists. Uh, it makes me shiver. I know it wants to spread, it aims for my whole body, it wants to completely take over me. It wants me to lose control. It has a bad, dark intention.... There is such despair in me, such utter loss of control, such helplessness. I must hide, I am going far, far away in my mind, I cannot bear this.... I feel like I want to explode, I feel like a bomb inside. Yet I have never told anybody. Who will understand the memory of a small girl now that I am nearly 50 years old? People will think I am crazy ...
Excerpt from a vivo-documented NET testimony, during therapy with a 49-year-old female survivor of childhood sexual abuse, 2003

Loneliness and social isolation are recurring themes among survivors. Unable to talk about the horrors of the past, unable to even comprehend "this other side, this crazy side" in oneself, the feelings become a part of, and seem to control, the behavior of this new and altered person. As one woman describes her experiences:

Even now many years later the pictures of this day keep coming back to my mind. I look at normal people, like a teacher or a friend, and suddenly the face of the perpetrator appears. Then I get angry and aggressive and try to hurt the person. I throw things and get violent. Sometimes I find myself sitting in strange places, like on top of the roof crying and I have no idea how I got there. It is as if there are two personalities living inside me. One is smart and kind and normal, the other one is crazy and violent. I try so hard to control this other side of me. But I fail. Sometimes I feel tears running down my cheek and I wonder why ... I have never told anybody what had happened to me during that day and even my father does not know what goes on in my mind and body when I get out of control. This is why I always feel a distance to everybody around me. People don't understand why I act strange sometimes, and I cannot tell them.... When I saw children playing and being happy I had to cry because I thought I could never do something like that again.
Excerpt from a vivo-documented NET testimony, during therapy with a 13-year-old Somali child survivor, 2003

From an outsider's perspective, it might seem that *narration* and *trauma* are radically opposed and mutually exclusive, as the people suffering these crimes are in too much pain, incapacitated by their enigmatic memory code, to share their stories. However, these two concepts are intimately connected. The atrocities cannot remain buried forever, and eventually the victim will be compelled to speak. It is this dichotomy that creates the foothold for this approach and this work.

After the war, for ten years I didn't speak, I was not a witness, for ten years ... and I was waiting for ten years, really.... I was afraid of language. Oh, I knew for ten years I would do something: I had to tell the story. One day, I visited an old Jew.... He sat down in his chair, and I in mine, and he began weeping. I have rarely seen an old man weep like that. I didn't know what to do. We stayed there like that, he weeping and I closed in my own pain. And then, at the end, he simply said, "You know, maybe you should talk about it...." In that year, the tenth year, I began my narrative.

Excerpt from an interview in 1996 with the Nobel Peace Prize laureate and survivor of Auschwitz Concentration Camp Elie Wiesel (Wiesel, 1996).

Speechlessness versus the wish and fear to disclose the events forms the central dialectic of psychological trauma. A naturally occurring conflict exists between wanting to deny the horrible events and feeling the urge to scream out the extent of the atrocities. Regaining one's dignity as well as finding truth in implicating the perpetrator are both fundamental to one's internal process of healing.

Not feeling understood becomes another major hurdle for some victims. The belief lives within that others will never be able to share their experience. Here is one person's testimony to this:

It is not because I cannot explain that you won't understand, it is because you won't understand that I can't explain.

Wiesel (1996)

If this core dynamic of *not feeling understood in the incommunicability* is not recognized, treatment is in vain. Previous approaches to healing and overcoming traumatization have tried to address this problem with different strategies, which may not have recognized these issues. By putting words to the trauma, victims are empowered to overcome their sense of speechlessness and lack of explicit memory. However, clinical intervention techniques are not sufficient. Trauma has societal and political dimensions, as do talking about the experiences, the terror, the torture, and the abuse. Victims may feel silenced because of the far-reaching political implications that verbalizing the abuse might have. This extends to mental health professionals as well, who may feel discomfort or overwhelmed while listening to stories that demonstrate a gross violation of human rights.

The ordinary response to atrocities is to banish them from consciousness. Denial, repression, and dissociation operate on a social as well as an individual level.... Far too often secrecy prevails, and the story of the traumatic event surfaces not as a verbal narrative but as a symptom. Remembering and telling the truth about terrible events are prerequisites both for the restoration of the social order and for the healing of individual victims.

J. L. Herman (1992b)

It is precisely these sociopolitical aspects of healing that need to be explicitly addressed. Only through an externalization of the feelings, abuse, and distrust, will true healing occur. Postconflict peace and reconciliation hinge both on a willingness of members of society to open their eyes to the abuse, and on the mental health of the individual. Narrative exposure therapy (NET) serves to address both the health of the individual, as well as society, based on the philosophy that these systems are inherently interrelated.

Given this theoretical foundation, NET works at the level of the individual by encouraging the telling of the trauma story and by reliving the past traumatic sceneries within an imaginative exposure design (see Foa, & Rothbaum, 1998). The goal is to allow for the modification of the *fear network* co-constructed by traumatic and stressful events (Lang, 1984, 1993; Schauer & Elbert, 2010). Thus NET weaves *hot implicit memories* into the story unfolded by *cool declarative memories* (see Elbert & Schauer, 2002; Metcalfe, & Jacobs, 1999). In this way, intrusive recollections and fragments are integrated into their original context, and a consistent autobiographical narrative develops. Part of the process is similar to that of creating a legal testimony. The logic of this part follows the testimony therapy procedure, as developed by Lira and Weinstein in Chile under the Pinocet regime (Cienfuegos & Monelli, 1983).

As narratives are an integrative part of every culture, NET is a culturally universal intervention for the reduction of traumatic stress symptoms in survivors of serious and repeated life-threatening events, such as organized violence, torture (see Amnesty International, 2003, and United Nations, 1984, for a definition for 'torture'), war, rape, civil trauma, and childhood abuse. NET is a form of exposure that encourages traumatized survivors to tell their detailed life history chronologically to a skilled counselor or psychotherapist who will record it, read it back, and assist the survivor with the task of integrating fragmented traumatic memories into a coherent narrative. Describing personal experiences in detail facilitates an internal visual recollection of, and thus exposure to, traumatic memories. Originally developed for survivors of multiple and complex forms of trauma who come from diverse backgrounds and who live in unsafe situations, often under conditions of continuous trauma, narrative exposure serves not only therapeutic purposes but also a social and political agenda. While NET is treating survivors through the narrative process, it is also simultaneously documenting violations of child rights and human rights.

Overall, this manual was written with the goal of integrating psychological rehabilitation of trauma survivors with issues of human rights and dignity on social, academic, and political levels. This work bridges the gap between science and fieldwork. It is aimed at mental health practitioners who work in the field (crisis regions, postconflict settings) as well as those individuals working in clinics, human rights organizations, public health institutions, and academic settings. At the same time, this manual is also written such that it is available to engaged members of the general public. Since story-telling, oral tradition, and verbal expression are concepts shared among all of humankind, NET can be tailored to any culture.

Based on scientific evidence from various disciplines (clinical psychology, neuropsychiatry, neuroscience, public health, and refugee studies), NET has been compiled and successfully field tested (e.g., Hensel-Dittmann, in press; Bichescu, Neuner, Schauer, & Elbert, 2007; Neuner, Schauer, Elbert, & Roth, 2002; Neuner, Schauer, Klaschik, Karunakara, & Elbert, 2004b; Neuner et al., 2008; Ruf et al., 2010; Schaal, Elbert, & Neuner, 2009; Schauer et al., 2006). Among other things, its applicability and efficacy for survivors of violence have been demonstrated under a variety of conditions such as refugee camps/settlements, national or local emergencies or crises, and in European and American outpatient clinic settings (for review, see Robjant & Fazel, 2010).

In sum, the core intention of creating NET has been to form a method of psychological treatment that will simultaneously heal while directly contributing to the fight against violence, abuse, maltreatment, torture, and persecution. The primary elements are thus threefold: healing of the individual, healing from violence committed against children and women or against one's ethnic or cultural group, and reconciliation from violence.

> Look, you must speak.
> As poorly as we can express our feelings, our memories, but we must try.
> We have to tell the story as best as we can.
> We cannot guarantee success, but we must guarantee effort.
>
> In truth, I have learned something:
> Silence never helps the victim. It only helps the victimizer....
> If I remain silent, I poison my soul.
>   Wiesel (1996)

Throughout this process, witnesses and survivors of civil child rights abuse and severe human rights vi-

olations are invited to work through their traumatic memories while narrating and testifying to the details. This practice enables the processing of painful emotions and the reconstruction of clear contingencies of dangerous and safe conditions, generally leading to significant emotional recovery. If the survivor agrees, the documents (testimonies) that result from this therapy can also be used directly for prosecution of human rights violations or for awareness-raising purposes to counteract societal forgetfulness and denial.

Traditional means of assessing and narrating human experience have failed to encompass and account for trauma, and yet it is necessary to speak about these events if we are to heal their rupture of personal lives and history. But how can we tell these stories? What is the consequence of testifying to that horror? What is the effect of bearing witness to such testimony?

> Now we recognize our duty to tell the full story, however painful,... the survivors need to come forward after all these years of silence...The silence that had been both a trap and a sanctuary for many survivors.

Dori Laub, child survivor of the Holocaust and clinical professor of psychiatry at Yale University and the Fortunoff Video Archive for Holocaust Testimonies at Yale (personal communication)

As a result, victims of violence are offered the chance to claim justice through documentation. From this, an important step may result. The violence is no longer completely senseless; an element of meaning is given to their terrifying experiences and the healing process. NET's explicit societal and political orientation and goal, enforcing the UN Declaration of Child Rights and Human Rights, has proven to be a significant asset in many ways. Human rights groups, courts of law or international criminal tribunals, or courts of law that rely on the validity of the data given by survivors can profit from the completeness of a victim's report. Advocacy activities, carried out on behalf of one's own people, also may be based on testimonial evidence provided by NET. But most of all, it is a documentation of a person's life, a memory that will be preserved and that can be passed on to children and grandchildren.

Based on our own experiences and observations of NET in practice, we have concluded that it is indeed possible that NET has empowering consequences on both individual and societal levels. Striving for appropriate mental health services for trauma victims turns out to be anything but a "luxury," especially in resource-poor, conflict-ridden countries (Schauer & Schauer, 2010). Many survivors suffering from disorders of extreme stress are unable to perform activities crucial to survival, such as creating viable economic and social living conditions for themselves and their families. Victims may be suffering from intrusions and nightmares, their physical health may be deteriorating, and feelings of worthlessness and suicidal ideations are likely to be increasing. Lives of trauma survivors are often characterized by hopelessness, poverty, and the inability to fulfill their societal roles. After treatment, it has been shown that survivors have been able to return to work, tend to their fields, and reengage in social and intimate relationships. With this, the process of individual and communal recovery is able to begin. Therefore, trauma treatment is a key link between an individual's mental health and those societal factors such as community and economic development.

Healing deep-seated antagonism or changing ideologies of antagonism through various types of interactive conflict resolution procedures can contribute to [reconciliation].... Members of each group can describe the pain and suffering of their group at the hands of the other.... They can grieve for themselves.... They can begin to grieve for the other as well. Members of each group can acknowledge the role of their own group in harming the other. Mutual acknowledgement of responsibility can lead to mutual forgiving. Healing from trauma, which reduces pain, enables people to live constructive lives, and reduces the likelihood of violence by victims and thus a continuing cycle of violence.

Staub (1998)

If it is indeed true that remembering and narrating the truth about terrible events are prerequisites for both healing of the individual victim as well as restoration of the social order and perhaps even reconciliation, postconflict peace, and economic development (Herman, 1992b), then why would we share the "conspiracy of silence?" At times it seems that we sometimes use the survivors feelings of incommunicability as an excuse not to hear their horrible stories. Here is one victim's voice that wants to encourage us:

The enemy wanted to be the one who speaks, and I felt, I still feel, we must see to it that the victim should be the one who speaks and is heard. Therefore, all my adult life, I always try to listen to the victim....
Be sensitive in every way possible. There is nothing more exciting than to be a sensitive person.

Because then you listen....
Of course it hurts. Sensitivity is painful. Think of those that you have to be sensitive to. Their pain is greater than yours.

Wiesel (1996)

There are fundamental issues that continue to arise as we conduct this work. For instance, am I convinced that it is good for the survivor to be exposed again to the traumatic memories? Will it contribute to healing, or cause more pain and disturbance? Do I want to hear these stories? What do I do about the fear I have listening to these stories? Searching for answers, we honor the victims' voices:

If you had seen such things that I went through, you'll never forget. Before I had told my story, the horrible experiences felt like wounds in my body that didn't want to heal. I was always sad. I didn't know what could help. The pictures were always there and I was shaking with fear, so I wasn't able to dig in the fields. Because of the pain I couldn't find the words. Only pieces of speech. Then you came and were not afraid to listen to me. To hear all of it. I never thought anybody could bear hearing this. Now I hold the story in my heart and on the paper in my hands. I cannot read, but my children will finally know what has happened, what enables them to fight for peace. Because I went through the pain, I got my past back. Now my heart is free....
Excerpt from a vivo-documented NET testimony with a 35-year-old female survivor of the Sudan Genocide, 2000

There are unique advantages to working through and documenting the biography of a person's entire life as is done in NETherapy. First of all, the treatment allows reflection on the person's entire life in retrospect. This will enable a person to realize how interwoven the elements of the largely implicit emotional network of the relevant experiences and events are – its attached positive and negative feelings. A new sense of perceived identity may emerge: "who am I" at present and "who was I" when trauma struck me. An inner process of understanding and realization of the origin and perception of one's feelings, thoughts, and behavioral patterns is initiated. Moreover, personal resources and strengths assembled throughout the lifespan ("flowers") can be uncovered and validated. Safe engagement and detailed unfolding of emotional networks will allow for integration: The meaning of interrelated configurations of life will be appreciated, and associated incidents rise to consciousness, a process creating a sense of one's "fateful" course of life. Insights about the past fall into place, so the implications and wishes for the future begin to show. The therapist, mental health expert, or trauma counselor is tasked to offer secure and personal bonding, while being fully present as a counterpart and listener, bearing witness, honoring, and respecting the survivor and every piece of her or his life as it has happened and as it keeps unfolding moment by moment.

2 Theoretical Background

2.1 Traumatic Stress

2.1.1 Traumatic Events

What we call trauma in colloquial language does not correspond well to the definition provided within the fields of clinical psychology and psychiatry. Trauma does not just refer to any breakdown in coping strategies in the face of difficult life events. Trauma means a cut into the soul as a result of a horrifying experience (see also Elbert & Schauer, 2002, for a brief outline of the concept). The wound may persist as a crippling disease with its core conceptualized as posttraumatic stress disorder (PTSD). The term *trauma* originally comes from Greek and means "injury or wound." It was first used in the field of medicine to describe bodily injury, such as with emergency medicine (physical trauma after an accident) or neurology (traumatic brain injury). Later, psychiatrists suggested that extremely stressful, typically life-threatening events could be considered traumatic, as those events could contribute to the onset of mental and subsequently also physical disorders, even without any physical injury. Trauma thus becomes the "wound of the soul." Consequently, the behavior, perception, and self-report of a specific symptom pattern as well as methods for examining survivors' brain functioning and structure became tools for "viewing" the mental injury. We will see in the next chapter how those survivors of trauma who still suffer from the impacts of the events also experience severe emotional pain when reminded of the event. Quite naturally, they try hard to avoid such reminders and to suppress related feelings. This is analogous to someone who has had a physical injury and avoids further pain by not moving or touching the injured part of the body.

Traumatic events are characterized by extraordinary circumstances and by the presence of distinct physiological alarm and defense responses in the victims when they do occur. Traumatic events are not just bad experiences that cause people to suffer. They are noted for the quality of the impact they have on human beings. These oftentimes life-threatening events can have a horrifying impact, regardless of whether the person was directly affected or whether the person simply witnessed the event happening to someone else. Both situations can be equally traumatizing; especially when the event happens to someone close, such as a family member or a loved one. We can classify traumatic experiences into two types: man-made disasters and natural disasters. Examples of traumatic events caused by other humans are exposure to combat, rape, torture, witnessing a massacre or mass killing, being held prisoner of war, or experiencing catastrophes such as airplane crashes or severe car accidents. Natural disasters classified as trauma may include floods, earthquakes, hurricanes, or volcanic eruptions. In contrast, experiences of loss, such as losing a business, or of bereavement, such as caring for an elderly parent, are not considered traumatic. Neither would viewing a horrifying movie or reading a violent book qualify as a *traumatic experience in adults*. Adult observers are constantly aware that movies are not real and therefore do not panic, in a state of alarm.

Even extremely stressful events are considered traumatic only when the victim or the eyewitness enters a physiological *alarm state* during the event, and the individual feels terrified or helpless or both. In this case, a cascade of responses in the body and mind is triggered which, when frequently reexperienced, will damage both the mind and the body. The stressful event is then called a traumatic one. This cascade involves a series of very rapid changes in body and brain mediated by neural activity, hormones, and changes in immune function, which affect all organs and include increased heart rate, muscle tone, blood flow, and metabolism; digestion is put on hold and resources are withdrawn from the immune system.

> **Summary   What is trauma?**
>
> *Psychological trauma* is the experience and psychological impact of events that are life-threatening or include a danger of injury so severe that the person is horrified, feels helpless, and experiences a psychophysiological alarm response during and shortly following the experience.

2.1.2 Stress and the Defense Cascade

The body, including the brain, has the ability to deal with danger in a flexible and adaptive way. In contrast to homeostasis, i.e., the organism's ability to maintain a steady internal state, there is considerable flexibility in the adjustment to stressors that range from physical deprivation (cold, noise, deprivation of food and of sleep, etc.) to the real or imagined fear-provoking situations that trigger an alarm response or a "shutdown" process, and thus may result in corresponding disorders of the trauma spectrum. Mammals including humans choose from an arsenal of attack and defense armaments to counter negative impact (McEwen, 2002; Schauer & Elbert, 2010). Even with minor cues, the brain can activate any appropriate alternative from the flight-fight-freeze-faint defense cascade. A coherent sequence of six defense responses that escalate as a function of proximity to danger and threat has been established by evolutionary biology and psychophysiology alike: freeze, flight, fight, fright, flag, and faint (Schauer & Elbert, 2010). First, the freezing (orienting response) facilitates a "stop-look-listen" perception and evaluation of the threat. Pavlov (1927) referred to it as "Shto Eta" (what is it?) – a reflex that turns the sensory systems to the source of stimulation and that can be viewed as a collection of bodily responses that assist in processing the stimulus further, such as papillary dilation, a drop in skin resistance, and a transient drop in heart rate. If the stimulus is perceived as a threat, an alarm response is initiated, with sympathetic arousal and adrenal release that enables the organism to counter danger (heart rate acceleration, blood pressure elevation, and vasoconstriction) – i.e., to flee or fight. It should be noted that highly aversive stimuli that appear close to the organism do not elicit an orienting response but rather a defensive reflex. For example, a very intense (say, 100 dB) noise with a short rise time, by its physical nature is likely to be from a nearby threat and elicits a startle response – pupils constrict and heart rate increases. This defensive reflex includes responses that assist in "blocking out" the event. The peritraumatic panic reaches its maximum in the fright response (tonic immobility), which may enhance survival when there is no more perceived possibility of escaping or winning a fight (direct physical contact with the perpetrator), finally leading to parasympathetic dominance (bradycardia, drop in blood pressure, and vasodilation) which may, in extreme cases, result in a

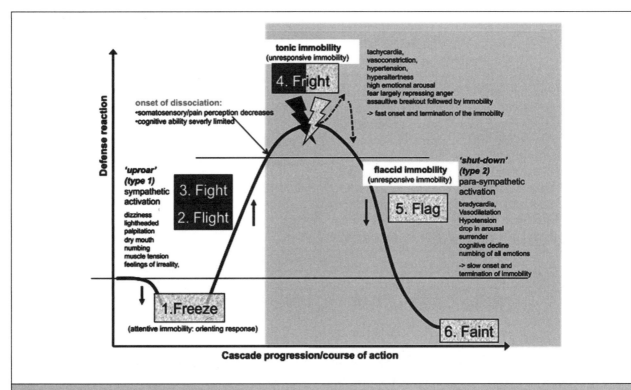

Figure 1. Schematic illustration of the defense cascade as it progresses along the course of different actions. The "uproar" sympathetic arousal reaches a maximum at the fright stage, eventually superseded by the onset of dissociative "shut down" (gray area). During life threat, not every stage of the defense cascade is necessarily passed through by the individual. The actual sequence of trauma-related response dispositions carried out in an extremely dangerous situation depends on several factors: The defense reactivity is organized to account for ability to defend oneself (chances to win a fight) of the threatened individual – i.e., the appraisal of the threat by the organism in relation to its own power to counteract (age, sex, physical condition, defensive abilities, etc.) and, not least, the threat specifics (type of threat, type and speed of approach, context, threat involving blood loss, etc.). In addition, a particular response may be classically conditioned and thus depend on previous experiences with threatening events. Adapted by permission from "Dissociation following traumatic stress: Etiology and treatment" by Maggie Schauer and Thomas Elbert, *Zeitschrift für Psychologie/Journal of Psychology, 218,* 109–127 (doi: 10.1027/0044-3409/a000018). © 2010 Hogrefe Publishing.

vasovagal fainting (-like) response (absence of efferent motor commands and functional deafferentation; Figure 1). The actual sequence of trauma-related response dispositions carried out in an extremely dangerous situation depends on the appraisal of the threat by the organism in relation to its own power to act (e.g., age, sex), as well as the perceived characteristics of the threat/perpetrator.

The cascade of these responses to stress is directed by four bodily systems (overview Elbert & Rockstroh, 2003; McEwen, 2002; Teicher, Andersen, Polcari, Anderson, & Navalta, 2002). The hippocampus is primarily responsible for functions associated with the build-up of memory, and the hypothalamic-pituitary-adrenal (HPA) axis is the elite force of the defense cascade and involved in the feedback regulation of cortisol, a stress hormone secreted by the adrenal gland. A second axis involves the amygdala (related to the development and processing of emotions), locus coeruleus, adrenal gland, and sympathetic nervous system, all crucial for directing blood flow, increasing awareness, and mobilizing the corresponding defense response. A third, less-explored axis involves the vasopressin-oxytocin peptides. Finally, in addition to these three axes, the immune system is involved in adaptive and maladaptive responses (see Segerstrom & Miller, 2004, for an overview): short-lasting acute and naturalistic stressors are associated with adaptive up-regulation of some, but down-regulation of other, parameters of immunity, while chronic stressors lead to immune suppression. All of these systems – when functioning properly – help us to deal with crisis. They are also involved in the stress-protective effect of positive social interaction, while, in turn, a dysregulated metabolism of specific biological systems may be associated with clinical disorders.

When unremitting stress forces the three axes of stress response to tilt in one direction, the result can be anything from a long-lasting head cold to depression. When tilted the other way, toward a flattening of the rhythm of stress hormones, undesirable consequences may be abdominal fat, loss of muscle mass, and mental ailing. When the danger is over, the stress response shuts down – at least in wild animals. Humans, however, seem to be unique in that they can keep the HPA axis going indefinitely. The stress hormones ultimately make their way back to the brain, affecting both behavior and health. The various stages of the defense cascade have evolved to allow adequate responding, such as running for escaping acute danger or dissociative responding or even fainting, when a predator has come too close, something invasive enters the body

(i.e., penetration of sharp objects), or contamination with bodily fluids is impending. However, a flight-fight response, as well as fainting, may be inappropriate in a modern human – after, e.g., a traffic accident or a bomb attack. Still, the same physiological responses (such as the supply of additional blood and oxygen to muscles, etc.) may be activated in the face of modern stressful stimuli, which cannot be attacked, or escaped by running away. Prolonged stress with its permanent initiation of the warding off stress will turn the adaptive physiological responses into maladaptive disease in the form of aches and pains, loss of appetite, or overeating. When repeated activation of the memories keep the defense responses activated, organs, including the brain, will be damaged.

Increasing evidence suggests that the brain is affected in various ways by stressful environments and experiences (Bremner, 2002). Two prime targets for stress hormones in the brain are the hippocampus and the amygdala. It is well established that acute elevations of adrenal stress hormones (catecholamines and glucocorticoids) enhance memory consolidation of emotionally arousing, contextual (hippocampus-dependent) information in a dose-dependent manner in animals (Roozendaal, de Quervain, Ferry, Setlow, & McGaugh, 2001) and humans (Buchanan & Lovallo, 2001; Cahill, Prins, Weber, & McGaugh, 1994). These enhancing effects of stress hormones are mediated by structures within (the basolateral nucleus of) the amygdala (Cahill, Babinsky, Markowitsch, & McGaugh, 1995; McGaugh, 2002). Whereas the support of stress hormones might be adaptive, whenever lasting memories of vital information (e.g., dangerous situations) have to be established, this mechanism may become maladaptive in conditions of extreme stress, when persistent and intrusive memories of a traumatic event promote the development of trauma-related disorders. However, acute elevations of glucocorticoids not only have enhancing effects on memory consolidation, but also impairing effects on memory retrieval (de Quervain, Roozendaal, & McGaugh, 1998; de Quervain, Roozendaal, Nitsch, McGaugh, & Hock, 2000; Roozendaal, Griffith, Buranday, de Quervain, & McGaugh, 2003). Furthermore, chronic glucocorticoid excess can lead to disruption of brain synaptic plasticity, atrophy of dendritic processes, and reduced neuronal ability to survive a variety of coincident insults (Sapolsky, 1999). Moreover, perinatal stress changes the HPA axis, delays cognitive and emotional development, and may impair avoidance learning for the rest of a person's life (Bock, Helmeke, Ovtscharoff, Gruß, & Braun, 2003; Meaney, Aitken, van Berkel, Bhatnagar, & Sapolsky, 1988; Teicher et al., 200Thus, stressful experiences differentially activate a variety of responses designed by evolution to counter danger. The different chemical messengers may cause deficits in hippocampus-based learning and memory, and their effects on the amygdala and the medial prefrontal and cingulate cortex may lead to impaired inhibition of fear responses. As a result, emotional and autobiographic memory may become fragmented (see Section 2.2). In addition, repeated or chronic exposure to traumatic stress may result in long-term dysregulation of these systems, leading to impaired functioning and to symptoms of stress-related disorders such as hyperarousal, dissociation, flashbacks, avoidance, and depression.

When confronted with trauma reminders, survivors typically "replay" their original response of the traumatic event (e.g., Keane, Zimering, & Caddell, 1985; Schauer & Elbert, 2010). When the original threat has triggered a fight/flight response, a corresponding alarm response with high emotional arousal and sympathetic responding may be elicited by the reminding cues. However, if a parasympathetically dominated shutdown was the prominent peritraumatic response to the traumatic incident, comparable dissociative responses may dominate responding to subsequently experienced threat and may also reappear when the traumatic memory is reactivated during therapy. The current concept of PTSD does not distinguish whether the reminder of the traumatic experiences results in a fight–flight alarm, an "uproar" or in a dissociative block, a shutdown with a subsequent excessive vagal tone. For the therapist, however, it is mandatory to note if the physiological responding during exposure is dominated by high emotional arousal or by a dissociative responding. To understand responding during trauma-focused treatment, it is thus necessary to understand the response repertoire humans have when confronted with various forms of threat to their lives (Figure 1).
Patients who respond to trauma with numbing, freezing, dissociation, or even fainting would be predicted to produce a muted or reduced psychophysiological response when recalling the event. Intrusions can be understood as repetitive displays of fragments of the event, which then elicit a corresponding combination of hyperarousal and dissociation, depending on the dominant physiological response during the threat.

We have suggested that repeated experience of traumatic stress may produce at least two major subtypes of clinical symptom profiles, depending on the physiological responding during the exposure (Schauer & Elbert, 2010): Those patients who showed (mainly) sympathetic activation in response to the stressor show little sign of dissociation and passive avoidance during exposure treatment, whereas those who went down the whole defense cascade via fright to fainting, which leads to parasympathetic dominance during the trauma, will produce a corresponding replay of physiological responding when reminded. The latter condition requires the management of dissociative stages (fright and faint) during treatment. Although each patient could be located in a two-dimensional space, e.g., with cumulative peritraumatic sympathetic and parasympathetic arousal as axes, we will, for the sake of simplicity, note that two subtypes appear in this two-dimensional space: Those who only showed repeated sympathetic arousal and those who also produced strong vagal responses at least in response to some traumatic stressors. We will call these two presumed subtypes "uproar-PTSD" (sympathetic-action PTSD) and "shutdown-PTSD" (vagal-dissociative PTSD).

An evolutionary perspective suggests, that shutdown enables survival in the following situations:
- When the organism is in direct and close encounter with a dangerous perpetrator, e.g., when there is skin contact;
- in the presence of body fluids with danger of contamination, e.g., blood or sperm;
- when bodily integrity is already injured, or in the face of impending or enforced invasion, e.g., sexual penetration, sharp objects (e.g., teeth or knife) at the skin, or medical procedures.

These situations require physiological adaptations, including immobility and analgesia for pain (in order to "play possum," avoid tearing tissue, pretend entire submission; for details, see Schauer & Elbert, 2010), and with them, "switches" in consciousness, information processing, and behavior, which are perceived as strange because they are outside the range of ordinary experiences.

2.1.3 Violence: The Major Source of Traumatic Stress

Forms of Violence
Violence appears in different forms. Prominent classifications of violence are defined according to context (Derriennic, 1971). A major dimension for qualifying types of violence rests on the degree of organization. Examples of unorganized types of violence include assaults, domestic violence, sexual abuse, and other violent crimes against individuals. Organized violence includes wars, armed conflict, political persecution, and any other systematic violation of human rights. Political motives provide the context for a more sys-

tematic order of organized or state-sponsored violence, which include torture, massacres, hand-to-hand combat, crimes against humanity, and bombardments. Organized violence is not a psychological crisis, such as a pervasive or chronic mental health issue like schizophrenia would be. It is important to be aware of the political context of war and torture and to comprehend the meaning of organized violence for individuals and society. Similarly, it is important to acknowledge the implications of domestic violence and abuse for the life of an individual survivor.

Survivors of Organized Violence

An obvious consequence of organized violence is that many people have to flee from their region of origin because of war or persecution. Figures released by the UN refugee agency for 2009 show that some 43.3 million people were forcibly displaced worldwide – the highest number of people uprooted by conflict and persecution since the mid-1990s. No matter where refugees or internally displaced people flee to after war and persecution, most exiles are not safe or accommodating (Karunakara et al., 2004). Many reports indicate that initial receptions by host government authorities and humanitarian agencies are impersonal and threatening, and that refugees assume roles of dependency and helplessness (Doná & Berry, 1999). While development of social networks, family reunions, and permanent settlements do occur (Castles & Miller, 1993), harsh living conditions, continued anxiety about forced repatriation, and uncertainties regarding resettlement can cause considerable stress for the refugees (Cunningham & Cunningham, 1997). Host country refugee policies are often dictated by domestic concerns, usually of a foreign policy nature, and not necessarily determined by security and protection concerns or by the wishes of host communities in receiving countries (Tandon, 1984). There are many reports that refugee camps and internal displacement camps breed violence, and people are often victims of violent acts perpetrated by the army, militias, humanitarian workers, and by their hosts (Malkki, 1995; Turner, 1999; UNHCR, 2002). For many women and children, the very acts of going to communal latrines (Martin, 1991) or collecting firewood and water can be extremely dangerous. In countries throughout the world, people are being detained and imprisoned arbitrarily without a fair trial. Many face torture or other forms of ill-treatment, as has been frequently documented by Amnesty International. They may be held in inhumane conditions that are cruel and degrading. Cumulative exposure to these stressors piles up and eventually results in PTSD, depression, and related disorders (see next section) (WHO/UNHCR, 1996).

Worldwide, millions of children under the age of 18 years have been, and continue to be, affected by armed conflict. They are recruited into government armed forces, paramilitaries, civil militia, and a variety of other armed groups. Often they are abducted at school, on the streets, or at home. Yet international law prohibits the participation in armed conflict of children aged under 18. Children routinely face other violence – at school, in institutions meant for their protection, in juvenile detention centers, and too often in their own homes. There are estimated to be between 100 million and 150 million street children in the world, and this number is growing. Of those, some 5–10% have run away from, or been abandoned by, their families.

Summary   What is organized violence?

Organized violence is violence with a systematic strategy. It is put into operation by members of groups with a centrally guided structure or political orientation (police units, rebel organizations, terror organizations, paramilitary, and military formations). It is targeted for continuous use against individuals and groups who have different political attitudes or nationalities, or who come from specific racial, cultural, and ethnic backgrounds. It is characterized by the violation of human rights and disregard of women's and children's rights. The consequences reach far into the future of a society.

Survivors of Family Violence

The quality of parent–child interactions predicts the risk for psychopathology over the lifespan
Michael J. Meaney (2008)

Family violence, also known as domestic abuse, spousal abuse, child abuse, or intimate partner violence, has many forms including physical aggression (hitting, kicking, biting, shoving, restraining, slapping, throwing objects), sexual violence, or threats thereof. Unemployment, poverty, substance abuse (e.g., excessive alcohol consumption), and mental illness of spouse/parent are important risk factors for family violence (De Bellis, 2002; Dube, Felitti, Chapman, Giles, & Anda, 2003; Jaffee, 2005; Margolin & Gordis, 2000). Childhood trauma has psychopathological and developmental consequences including adverse emotional, behavioral, and cognitive consequences (De Bellis, 2002). High levels of stress, fear, and anxiety are commonly reported by victims of domestic violence. Depression is also common, as victims are made to feel guilty for "provoking" the abuse, and are constantly subjected to verbal abuse or intense criticism. It is reported that 60% of victims meet the diagnostic criteria for depression, either during or after termination of the relationship, and have a greatly increased risk of suicidality (Barnett, 2001). In addition to depression, victims of domestic violence also commonly experience long-term anxiety and panic, and are likely to meet the diagnostic criteria for a Generalized Anxiety Disorder or Panic Disorder. The most commonly referenced psychological effect of domestic violence is PTSD (Vitanza & Vogel, 1995). Maltreatment of children, defined as neglect, physical abuse, sexual abuse, and emotional abuse (which includes witnessing domestic violence), has always been the most common cause of interpersonal trauma and PTSD in children and adolescents (De Bellis et al., 1999). Among other problems such as severe anxiety, depression, and externalizing behavior, from 10 victims of childhood abuse and neglect, about four develop PTSD (Widom, 1999). In clinically referred samples, the reported incidence rates of PTSD resulting from sexual abuse range from 42% to 90% (McLeer, Callaghan, Henry, & Wallen, 1994; McLeer et al., 1998) and are above 50% when arising from just witnessing domestic violence (Pynoos & Nader, 1989).

Children who grow up in an environment of violence and maltreatment later show severe forms of disorders of the trauma spectrum. Pathological levels of stress are thought to disrupt the normally integrative functions of mental activity, leading some aspects of experience to be segregated from conscious awareness. A number of studies have demonstrated significant associations between childhood physical or sexual abuse and dissociation (Dutra, Bureau, Holmes, Lyubchik, & Lyons-Ruth, 2009). Meta-analyses have confirmed the associations among infant disorganized attachment behavior, parental maltreatment, parental psychopathology, disturbed parent–infant interaction, and childhood behavior problems (Madigan et al., 2006). When intense and persistent stress occurs when the brain is undergoing enormous change, the impact may leave an indelible imprint on its structure and function (Matz et al., 2010; Teicher, et al., 2002). Especially childhood sexual abuse is a risk factor for the emergence of adult psychopathology such as depression (Andersen & Teicher, 2008), borderline personality disorder (Lieb et al., 2004; McLean, & Gallop, 2003), eating disorders (Schaaf & McCanne, 1994; Smolak & Murnen, 2002), somatization disorder (Farley & Keaney, 1997; Kinzl, Traweger, & Biebl, 1995; Morrison, 1989; Walker et al., 1992), and negative effects on physical health (Anda et al., 2005).

A recent prospective study (Widom, Czaja, & Paris, 2009) found that significantly more abused and/or ne-

glected children overall met the criteria for borderline personality disorder (BPD) as adults, compared with controls, as did physically abused and neglected children. Having a parent with alcohol/drug problems and not being employed full-time, not being a high school graduate, and having a diagnosis of drug abuse, major depressive disorder, and PTSD were predictors of BPD and mediated the relationship between childhood abuse/neglect and adult BPD.

Early stress or maltreatment is an important risk factor for the later development of substance abuse. There are windows of vulnerability for different brain regions when they are exposed to stress (Section 2.2.4). The following modifications in brain structure and function are designed to adapt the individual to cope with continuous adversity and deprivation. Even as an adult, the survivor will maintain a state of vigilance, hyperarousal, sympathetic activation, and suspiciousness to readily detect danger, and the potential to mobilize immediate aggression when threatened with danger or loss. Early childhood abuse and neglect lead individuals into social isolation, hostility, and depression and substance abuse, and foster the emergence of disease processes.

In war zones, children are often victims of both organized and family violence. The combination of these two forms of adversities potentiates the vulnerability for trauma-spectrum disorders (Catani et al., 2009, 2010).

Summary   What is familial violence?

Familial and domestic violence have many forms including physical aggression, sexual abuse, emotional neglect, verbal abuse, intimidation, and various forms of deprivation. Domestic and familial violence are common and thus often aggravate effects of other stressful experiences. Hence therapists should assess every client for these forms of violence. Survivors of early maltreatment and abuse often show a range of problems and severe symptoms of complex trauma. Compared with traumatic stressors experienced during adulthood, continuous and developmental trauma during development has even more serious consequences on the brain (see Section 2.2.4) and mind, and thus on the mental and physical well-being of the survivor.

2.1.4 The Concept of PTSD

The lasting pathological reactions to traumatic, stressful experiences are called posttraumatic symptoms. The prefix *post-* means "after" or "later" – so *post-traumat-*

ic means literally "after the injury" (of the soul). The study of the psychological consequences of traumatic events has a long tradition in psychiatry. In the 1970s, research studying the consequences of traumatic stress was stimulated by the finding that a large proportion of Vietnam veterans had major difficulties reintegrating into their prewar roles. At the same time, researchers influenced by the women's movement responded to the observation of severe psychological problems in rape victims and began research in this area.

The current definition of PTSD in the *Diagnostic and Statistical Manual of Mental Disorders,* fourth edition (DSM-IV) (APA, 1994, 1997; for the concept see Friedman, 2000) outlines six criteria that must be met at some level for a diagnosis of PTSD. They are as follows (refer also to the Summary Box):

(A) The first criterion refers to the *traumatic event.* PTSD can only be diagnosed when the symptoms are the result of some experienced or witnessed event that involved an actual or perceived threat to the life or physical integrity of the survivor or another person (A1). In addition, the immediate reaction of the victim must involve fear, terror, or helplessness (A2) – i.e., include an alarm response.

(B) The second criterion is related to *intrusive symptoms.* In the context of PTSD, intrusive symptoms describe the chronic reliving of the event. This may come in the form of nightmares while one is sleeping, or flashbacks that occur during waking hours. The phenomenon of reliving the event in the form of waking-hour flashbacks, which are accompanied by multiple sensory experiences (hearing the bombs, feeling the weight of the bodies) as well as the sense of being back in the traumatic situation seems to be unique to PTSD (Brewin, 2001).

(C) This third criterion relates to the *avoidance behavior* associated with PTSD. Contrary to the current classification, a factor analysis (a statistical procedure which groups like variables) of PTSD symptoms suggested the subdivision of avoidance symptoms into two different groupings (Foa, Riggs, & Gershuny, 1995). The first factor (or grouping) includes *active avoidance* of reminders of the traumatic event. For instance, one might avoid people and places that are associated with the event, or avoid talking or thinking about the event. The second factor relates to *passive avoidance* or *numbing.* These phenomena, which are also related to dissociation phenomena, include general emotional numbing as well as detachment from other people.

(D) The fourth criterion relates to a third group of symptoms. This group of symptoms consists of the *arousal symptoms* (Criterion D). These result from an overall elevated level of arousal, which may come in the form of sleeping and concentration difficulties, an exaggerated startle response, or the enduring feeling of threat.

Note: The symptoms of Criteria B-D in PTSD do not automatically disappear in survivors as the PTSD resolves itself, but may persist for a long time.

(E) Criterion E sets a time frame for PTSD, as the disturbance symptoms (Criteria B-D) (APA, 2000) must last for at least 4 weeks.

(F) Criterion F relates to the clinical significance of the disorder, as a remarkable reduction in day-to-day functioning is required for the diagnosis of PTSD. To decide whether the consequences of traumatic events classify as a mental disorder rather than adaptive behavior, it is important to study the level of functional impairment that is associated with PTSD in the current environment of the survivor. Breslau (2001) compared the level of impairment associated with PTSD and other mental disorders (mainly other anxiety disorders and depression) on several indicators, including current limitations in activities, missed work, self-assessed health, as well as desire to die. The PTSD patients presented with the worst outcome in respect to all criteria compared to both the individuals with other diagnoses and those without a diagnosis. A striking result from this study was that almost half (46%) of those who were diagnosed with PTSD reported that they had thought about suicide. Some 17% also reported completing a suicide attempt. PTSD also affects social functioning. Investigating the quality of intimate relationships of Vietnam veterans, Riggs and colleagues (Riggs, Byrne, Weathers, & Litz, 1998) found that 70% of veterans who had been diagnosed with PTSD were in relationships characterized by clinically significant levels of relationship distress; this rate was much lower among veterans without PTSD (30%). In particular, veterans with PTSD presented more aggression toward their intimate partners and were at increased risk for perpetrating domestic violence (Byrne & Riggs, 1996).

It is likely that these diagnostic criteria for PTSD and its variants will be somewhat different in the fifth edition of the DSM (DSM-V), which is due for publica-

Summary   DSM-IV criteria for PTSD

The six criteria for PTSD (*Diagnostic and Statistic Manual of Mental Disorders,* fourth edition [DSM-IV] of the American Psychiatric Association) (APA, 1994):
Criterion A1 = experiencing or witnessing a life-threatening "traumatic event." **Criterion A2** = subjective feelings of helplessness, fear, or horror during that event. **Criterion B** = reliving or reexperiencing of the traumatic event – "Intrusions." **Criterion** C = avoidance of reminders of the traumatic event – "Avoidance."
Criterion D = being overly aroused, alert, nervous – "Hyperarousal."
Criterion E = a minimum of 4 weeks suffering from these consequences.
Criterion F = severe problems in social, occupational, or other everyday functioning.
All criteria have to be fulfilled to diagnose posttraumatic stress disorder (PTSD).

tion in 2013. One controversial aspect concerns the DSM-IV Criterion A1 (Friedman, 2010). Evidence that PTSD does occur among people who have learned about traumatic exposure of a close friend or a loved one suggests that the "learned about" category will be retained as a criterion, possibly with a narrowing of the list of qualifying events such as homicide, gruesome death, grotesque details of rape, genocide, or violent abuse of a loved one. Criterion A2 is fulfilled in nearly all cases and therefore will be eliminated from the list.

Criterion C (avoidance/numbing) will be split in active avoidance and "negative cognitions and mood" as a new category. That will encompass the nonfear, dysphoric mood states associated with PTSD, such as guilt, shame, anger, and disgust. It will also cover negative cognitions such as self-blame and persistent negative expectations about oneself and the future. The category for hyperarousal and reactivity will probably be expanded to include behavioral and emotional indices of excessive arousal and reactivity, such as aggressive, reckless, and self-destructive behavior (along with insomnia, hypervigilance, startle, and cognitive impairment). The PTSD concept, with its dominant features of intrusive reliving and, hyperarousal reflects the 'uproar' side of the defense cascade (see 2.1.2): During sympathetic dominance, sensoric functioning and physiological excitement is heightened. However, some types of trauma (e.g., sexual abuse) result in a conditioned parasympathetic 'shut down' reaction with functional sensoric deafferentation. Those trauma survivors will not easily show intrusions which are required for the diagnosis

of PTSD (Schauer & Elbert, 2010). It can take years or decades until the first explicit intrusive memories appear. Nevertheless, those patients are severely traumatized and show many other symptoms of trauma spectrum disorders.

Summary   How does a traumatized person feel?

Traumatization means suffering from a memory of a traumatic experience that has happened in the past. Reexperiencing the traumatic event means that the survivor involuntarily relives this situation, either while awake in the form of flashbacks, or at night in the form of nightmares. Both are accompanied by intense feelings of fear and anger, often similar to the emotions that were experienced during the traumatic event itself. The body reacts in a stress response while remembering the event: The person's heart beats fast, they begin to sweat, and painful bodily sensations may arise. The memories may come back repeatedly no matter how much the person does not want to remember. Flashbacks also can be experienced in different ways. The person may know quite well that the flashback is just a memory and feel safe in the here and now, or the person may not realize it is just a memory and may feel an intense feeling of fear and lack of safety. The person may actually believe the traumatic situation is happening again. In rare cases, this can last for up to 10s of minutes. Some survivors describe the memories pulling them back into the past and that they are stuck in those moments of greatest fear. When nightmares occur, the survivor often awakes in a state of fear and can not go back to sleep again. Reexperiencing can be elicited by environmental cues, such as sounds or smells similar to those experienced during the traumatic event. Although the patient may not know exactly what triggered the memories, these same situations are often avoided in future. For instance, they may stop seeing certain people, stop going to certain places, or stop doing certain activities, all in an attempt to avoid reminders of the dreadful experiences. The patient may learn to be numb or to dissociate from reality, which may lead to a loss of loving feelings and of being able to feel close to people, even to their own spouse or children. The patient may lose hope or may feel the future has nothing to hold. At the same time, the heightened level of arousal (excitement) resulting from permanent or repeatedly triggered fear, leads to states of increased alertness and readiness to counter danger at any time. Patients may become mistrustful and suspect danger everywhere or may have difficulties focusing their attention on activities of daily living or listening to others. When asked what they have just heard, read or seen, they may be unable to tell you.

2.1.5 Psychosocial Problems and Comorbid Disorders in Adults and Children

Functional impairment that results from and often accompanies PTSD may be aggravated by symptoms that are not included in the DSM-IV diagnosis. These other symptoms may be related to comorbid mental disorders (disorders that occur simultaneously with PTSD, such as depression or anxiety; McFarlane, Atchison, Rafalowicz, & Papay, 1994). Epidemiological studies have found that one or more comorbid psychiatric disorders diagnosed in addition to PTSD occur in 80% of cases (Kessler, Sonnega, Bromet, Hughes, & Nelson, 1995). Table 1 lists the disorders that often exist in parallel with PTSD.

Comorbid disorders may occur independently as a result of the traumatic experience. For example, a victim may develop symptoms of depression following a traumatic loss. More often, however, the disorder is actually an extension of the core symptoms of PTSD. For instance, a victim who is experiencing vivid flashback episodes might experience a panic attack, indicative of panic disorder. Or, if someone feels detached and isolated from others, this person might abandon previous interests and hopes, start drinking or become clinically depressed. Another explanation for the comorbidity rates is that some underlying vulnerability present in an individual might increase the probability for that person to develop PTSD as well as other mental disorders.

In addition to experiencing psychosocial problems and mental health disorders, a child's normal healthy development may also be impaired. Factors such as altered memory function, frequent severe headaches, sleep disturbance, or loss of ability to concentrate may lead to a decline in school performance or difficulties in forming interpersonal relationships. In a survey of adolescents, Somasundaram (1993) found psychosocial problems and comorbid disorders as a consequence of these children being exposed to traumatic experiences during the war (Table 2).

In one international, epidemiological survey among Tamil children (Elbert et al., 2009), 57% of the children reported that traumatizing war experiences and the symptoms resulting from it interfered with their life. Social withdrawal, difficulties in leading a normal family life, and problems in school performance were most common. The greater the number of traumatic events reported, the greater the number of difficulties in social and emotional functioning reported by the child. Neuropsychological testing and school grades validated the outcome further and demonstrated the problem associated with this mental disorder. A psychological test of memory (the Rey-Osterrieth Complex Figure) revealed that nearly all children without PTSD scored perfectly, and were able to copy a figure by memory. However, interaction of PTSD diagnosis with recall shows that traumatized children are less able to perform well on this test and are unable to recall the different elements of the Rey Figure correctly. The recall score (% correctly recalled elements) dropped from 73% in the children without PTSD to 55% in those suffering from PTSD (Figure 2).

Clinical interviews in this study further revealed that depressive symptoms were frequent in children with PTSD. In response to questions relating to affective disorders, only 12% of the children without PTSD re-

Table 1. DSM-IV disorders frequently comorbid with PTSD		
Diagnosis	**Lifetime prevalence**	**Remarks**
Major Depression	48%	
Dysthymia	22%	
Generalized Anxiety Disorder	16%	
Simple Phobia	30%	
Social Phobia	28%	
Panic Disorder	12.6% vs. 7.3%	Women > men
Agoraphobia	22.4% vs. 16.1%	Women > men
Alcohol abuse/Dependence	51.9% vs. 27.9%	Men > women
Drug abuse/Dependence	34.5% vs. 26.9%	Men > women
Conduct Disorder	43.3% vs. 15.4%	Men > women
Adapted from Kessler et al. (1995).		

Table 2. Psychosocial problems in Tamil adolescents (n = 625)

Psychosocial problem	Percentage
PTSD	31
Somatization	32
Anxiety	34
Depression	29
Hostility	45
Relationship problems	34
Alcohol and drug misuse	7
Functional disability	35
Loss of memory	44
Loss of concentration	48
Loss of motivation	33

Adapted from Somasundaram (1993).

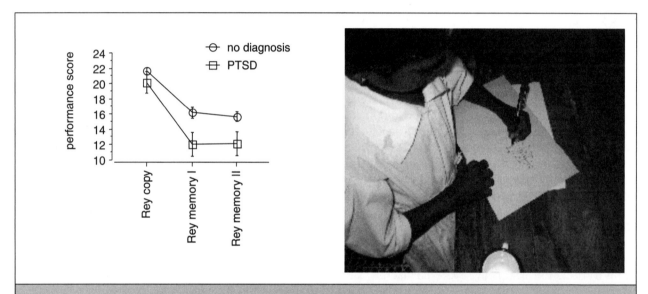

Figure 2. Children with and without PTSD can copy the Rey Figure equally well, but memory performance (right side: recall of the figure from memory) is better in children without PTSD (circles) than in those who present with PTSD (squares). Adapted from Child Abuse & Neglect, 33, Elbert et al. „Trauma-related impairment in children – A survey in Sri Lankan provinces affected by armed conflict", pp. 238-246, Copyright 2009, with permission from Elsevier.

ported symptoms of a mood disorder in comparison with 68% of those with PTSD, and more than 40% of the latter fulfilled the diagnosis for an affective disorder. The risk of suicide was 26% in the children who presented with PTSD versus 7% in children without PTSD. Somatic symptoms (physical illness–related symptoms) were also more frequently reported in children with PTSD than in those without PTSD. For instance, 81% of children with PTSD reported suffering from headaches during the last 4 weeks. In addition, children with PTSD had significantly lower school performance rates in key subjects compared with non-PTSD children (Elbert et al., 2009).

Often, children are also indirectly affected by trauma. Their parents' and caretakers' symptoms of PTSD, such as emotional numbing and avoidance, prevent normal emotional feelings and loving behavior toward their children. As a result, family members of a traumatized person are forced to operate within a domestic context in which intimacy is severely impaired. In many cases, tension, domestic violence, and substance abuse increase. Children are more likely to be abused or neglected as a consequence. Furthermore, severe traumatic experiences have multigenerational effects. Some evidence suggests there are higher rates of anxiety and depression in children of survivors compared with nontraumatized comparison groups. However, more rigorous scientific studies are needed to uncover the psychopathological consequences in the offspring of survivors.

PTSD and Drug Abuse

Drug use and abuse is part of any discussion about mental health and PTSD. Substance use – e.g., use of alcohol, cigarettes, marihuana, cocaine, heroin, amphetamines, khat, or banji seeds – is by far the most predominant cause of premature and preventable illness, disability, and death in most societies. Whereas abuse of, and dependence on, substances may in their own right bring suffering and physical sickness that require medical treatment, they often accompany other seemingly unrelated mental illnesses as well. PTSD patients tend to consume more drugs in an effort to reduce the mental pain associated with their symptoms; however, in the long-term, substance abuse only adds to the suffering, bringing its own mental and physical anguish. If drug abuse is found in children and adolescents, it is always a cry for help and as such should not be punished. It is of key importance to emphatically explore the reasons for such behavior, together with the troubled youngster. Traumatic events, but also suffering related to neglect or abuse during childhood years, are likely causes. A number of treatment programs exist that can reach substance abusers and their families. Successful trauma treatment, however, is necessary for these programs to work.

PTSD and Physical Illness

Since a long time there exist clinical observations and systematic studies, that the organism does not simply forget traumatic events: the 'body keeps the score' (van der Kolk, 1994). The relationship between stress and physical illnesses, in particular infectious diseases, has been well established and there are several assumptions about the immunological mechanisms that may be responsible for this effect (Kiecolt-Glaser et al., 2003). Given that PTSD is a chronic stressor for a person, it will exert its adverse effects on the health of the individual. PTSD patients show high physical morbidity with increased risk for a large number of diseases including cancer, coronary heart disease, and autoimmune disorders. In accordance with this finding, our group found that experiencing traumatic events leads to severe immunological alterations, e.g., a reduction in naïve cytotoxic and regulatory T cells, which can explain the increased risk for infections and autoimmune diseases, respectively (Sommershof et al., 2009). Exposure to trauma can also lead to problems with pain perception, pain tolerance, and chronic pain.

Vulnerability for PTSD

Epidemiological studies have shown that not everyone who experiences a traumatic event develops chronic PTSD; on the contrary, PTSD is the exception rather than the rule to a single traumatic exposure. The most adverse single event seems to be rape, as it leads to PTSD in about half of victims, followed by participation in war (two out of five individuals), and childhood abuse (more than one third) (Kessler et al., 1995). However, rape is usually not an isolated event, but often follows a history of earlier sexual abuse. There is a multitude of events. The same is true for war: Participation in armed conflict often means years of chronic stress with many traumatic experiences. And, as we detail below, the number of traumatic experiences is the main predictor for PTSD and also for its spontaneous remission.

Pretrauma vulnerability factors such as education, previous trauma, childhood adversity, psychiatric history, and family psychiatric history predicted PTSD consistently in several studies, but only to a surprisingly small extent. Factors operating during the event, such as trauma severity, or immediately after the event, such as lack of social support, seem to have stronger effect sizes, but still their explanatory power is small. The original conceptualization of PTSD was based on the implicit assumption that the traumatic event is the main agent for the development of PTSD (Yehuda & McFarlane, 1995). The idea was that traumatic events could cause PTSD in anyone regardless of pretrauma vulnerability.

While it can be doubted that there are single events that cause chronic PTSD in all victims, some studies show that a history of previous traumatic events increases the probability of developing PTSD after a subsequent event (Brewin, Andrews, & Valentine, 2000). We carried out a study that showed that the cumulative number of traumatic events experienced was the main predictor of PTSD among the war-affected Sudanese and Ugandan West-Nile populations. In the studied population, we found that every person who reported more than some 25 traumatic events in their lifetime met the criteria for PTSD. Nobody seems to be resilient at such a level of repeated threat (Neuner et al., 2004a; Schauer et al., 2003). This means that PTSD has a "building block" effect and that exposure to trauma and violence is cumulative or additive, contributing to the development of PTSD over time, given a high enough "dose" of trauma (Schauer et al., 2003). This building block effect has recently been replicated in different cultures and contexts: e.g., for samples of Rwandan genocide survivors by Schaal & Elbert (2006), for Rwandan and Somali refugees by

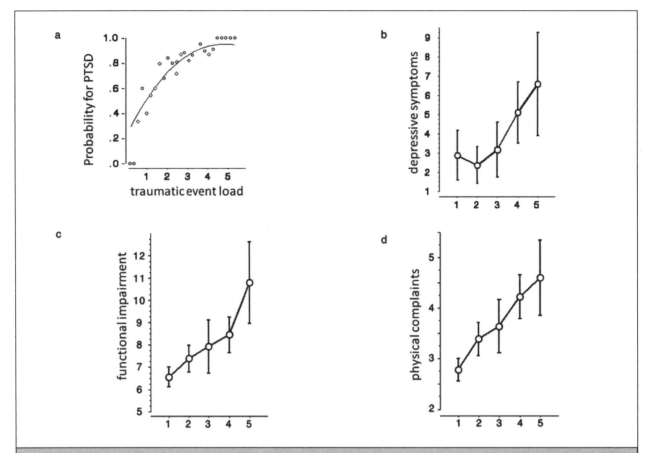

Figure 3. The probability of developing PTSD increases with cumulative experience of types of traumatic events experienced (figure 3a). Units on the abscissa correspond to classes of cumulative experiences of traumatic stressors. The full range is about 25 different types experienced, i.e., one unit corresponds to an exposure of five traumatic stressors. Circles indicate the observed average for PTSD for a particular event load. For those who have developed a PTSD, depressive symptoms, functional impairment, and physical diseases also become more likely with increasing exposure to traumatic stressors. Figure 3a: Data from survivors of the Rwandan genocide. Adapted from "The probability of spontaneous remission from PTSD depends on the number of traumatic event types experienced" by I. T. Kolassa, V. Ertl, S. Kolassa, L. P. Onyut, & T. Elbert, 2010, *Psychological Trauma: Theory, Research, Practice, and Policy, 2,* 169–174. Figures b-d: Data from a survey in Sri Lankan school children exposed to civil war. Adapted from "The psychological impact of child soldiering" by E. Schauer and T. Elbert, 2010, in E. Matz (Ed.), *Trauma rehabilitation after war and conflict* (pp. 311–360). New York, NY: Springer.

Onyut et al. (2009), and for Tamil children by Elbert et al. (2009) and Catani et al. (2010) (see also Figure 3.).

As mentioned above, a significant proportion of PTSD sufferers remit over time, even without treatment. Our data consistently not only showed that higher trauma exposure was associated with higher prevalence of current and lifetime PTSD but also with a lower probability of spontaneous remission from PTSD in a clear dose–response effect (Kolassa et al., 2010). Multiple studies have investigated the factors influencing remission from PTSD after single traumatic events. Unfortunately, previously experienced traumatic stress and exposure to violence, including domestic violence, has often not, or at least not properly, been assessed.

After motor vehicle accidents, higher initial symptom severity scores, new traumata to family members, more severe physical injuries, and unremitting physical injuries 4 months after the initial diagnosis were associated with lower rates of remission from PTSD 6 months after the initial diagnosis (Blanchard et al., 1997). A study of patients in primary care with PTSD found that remission during a 2-year follow-up was associated with lower comorbid anxiety disorders and higher psychosocial functioning at intake (Zlotnick et al., 2004). In a population of victims of physical and sexual assault, maintenance of PTSD was higher if the victim had held negative trauma-sensitive beliefs prior to the assault, if the victim experienced mental defeat or mental confusion during the trauma, or if the victim exhibited a negative appraisal of initial posttrauma symptoms or avoidance or safety-seeking as a maladaptive control strategy after the trauma (Dunmore, Clark, & Ehlers, 2001).

Culture and PTSD

There is no evidence for the hypothesis that the prevalence and validity of PTSD depends on cultural factors. Contrary to the statements that there is no universal trauma response, current research into the epidemiology of PTSD and the neurobiological mechanisms behind PTSD offer strong arguments for the theory that PTSD is a pathological consequence of traumatic events that occurs in all cultures. Obviously, this possibility to break the mind is an integral part of being human. There are studies of PTSD from all continents, and local experts from all continents have contributed to the research in this field.

Some people have argued that the transfer of Western concepts and techniques to war-affected societies in developing countries risks "perpetuating the colonial status of the non-Western mind" as every "culture has its own frameworks for mental health, and norms for help-seeking at times of crisis" (Summerfield, 1997, p. 1568; 2004). This argument is based on a clear distinction between Western Eurocentric cultures and other cultures in nonindustrialized countries. This distinction may seem to be straightforward, but it is not valid. Viewing culture as a particular civilization at a particular stage, there is always a wide diversity of attitudes, values, and habits, and neither frontiers between countries nor between the industrialized and nonindustrialized world can offer valid borderlines for cultural categories. The same is true for health and mental concepts. Many societies in developing countries have already chosen to adapt mental health concepts developed by Western psychology and psychiatry and prefer the corresponding treatment methods rather than, or in combination with, traditional healing. At the same time, in many rural areas in European countries, traditional healing techniques for physical and mental complaints have remained popular.

Those clinicians who emphasize the differences between cultures and advocate noninterference in cultures that are considered to be "traditional" use ethical arguments. Terms such as *culturally sensitive* are now included in mental health proposals and articles as a matter of political correctness. Even on moral grounds, it is not straightforward to favor the position of not interfering in cultural traditions, norms, and beliefs in psychosocial work. All cultures are constantly changing, and the idea that there are any societies that fully rely on traditional norms and have not been affected by the modern world is nothing more than the romantic view of Western minds. The consequences of not interfering in cultural norms would also include withholding knowledge about general scientific methods of objective assessment and evaluation from these cultures (see Neuner & Elbert, 2007, for further discussion).

There are considerable similarities and consistencies in the clinical manifestations of psychopathology across different refugee groups; these similarities and consistencies outweigh cultural and ethnic differences. Knowledge of this should lead us away from treating the mental health difficulties of refugees as something new and unusual while allowing us to focus attention on developing culturally sensitive assessment and treatment approaches to meet the special needs.

Garcia-Peltoniemi (1991)

It is these methods that have led to the development of treatment approaches that have proven to be effective and that have led to the identification of less successful or even harmful methods in many fields of healing and medicine. Withholding this knowledge from resource-poor countries might help to leave cultural norms untouched, but at the same time the global discrepancies in development and power remain unchanged. Protecting societies that are considered to be traditional from modern influences risks building cultural reservations of societies that remain dependent on the goodwill of the powerful countries.

There is now considerable knowledge about the epidemiology and validity of the PTSD concept in a wide variety of cultures. Until now, however, there have been few treatment studies, besides those performed by the humanitarian organization "vivo", that have evaluated the efficacy of different approaches in war-affected populations in developing countries. At this level of knowledge, it is an ethical obligation of psychosocial organizations to concentrate research on how the problem of mental health in these societies can be approached most effectively. The practice of many organizations in implementing large-scale psychosocial projects with nonevaluated treatment approaches is unacceptable. The alternative, however, is to demand more research instead of supporting a blanket rejection of current approaches in the field of mental health. What is necessary are empirically valid trauma-focused guiding principles for public mental health interventions for which evidence has been gathered. Such research is intended to bring awareness and action into a nearly neglected field of public health, human rights implementation, humanitarian intervention, development aid, policy making and funding; which will substantiate the thesis that a programmatic innovation is needed, rendering a paradigm shift inevitable (see Schauer & Schauer, 2010).

2.1.6 Complex PTSD

Until today, in the international manuals DSM and the *International Statistical Classification of Diseases and Related Health Problems,* 10th edition (ICD-10)

Summary Complex
I.   Alteration in regulation of affect and impulses A. Chronic affect dysregulation B. Difficulty modulating anger C. Self-destructive and suicidal behavior D. Difficulty modulating sexual involvement E. Impulsive and risk-taking behaviors
II. Alterations in attention or consciousness A. Amnesia B. Transient dissociative episodes and depersonalization
III. Somatization A. Digestive system B. Chronic pain C. Cardiopulmonary symptoms D. Conversion symptoms E. Sexual symptoms
IV. Alteration in self-perception A. Chronic guilt, shame, and self-blame B. Feelings of being permanently damaged C. Feeling ineffective D. Feeling nobody can understand E. Minimizing the importance of the traumatic event
V. Alterations in perception of the perpetrator (not needed for diagnosis) A. Adopting distorted beliefs B. Idealization of the perpetrator C. Preoccupation with hurting the perpetrator
VI. Alterations in relations with others A. Inability to trust B. Revictimization C. Victimizing others
VII.Alterations in systems of meaning A. Despair, hopelessness B. Loss of previously sustaining beliefs

(WHO, 1993), there is no settled diagnostic category for the type of continuous interpersonal trauma that goes along with conditioned shutdown reactions (Schauer & Elbert, 2010). Other than accidental single traumata, these repeated and overwhelming experiences, especially during childhood, modify the brain in structure and function to adapt individuals to cope with the high levels of stress and deprivation they may expect to encounter throughout the rest of their lives (Teicher, 2002). Already Herman (1992) has suggested differentiating between two different types of traumata, classifying the diversity of traumatic events according to their impact. Type I traumatic events are those events that lead to pathological consequences after a single exposure, such as a car accident or an isolated rape. The more severe Type II events include those that happen repeatedly over an extended time period, accounting for symptoms experienced by survivors of torture, childhood sexual abuse, or prisoner-of-war camps. In these cases, victims could foresee the next traumatic experience but could not influence the timing and had no way of escaping other than through dissociation of consciousness. This leads to comorbid problems and clinical symptoms in addition to, and beyond, the symptom triad of intrusion, avoidance, and arousal. As described before, enduring personality changes may occur (see ICD-10 F62.0). This "complex PTSD" was subsequently also called disorder of extreme stress (DES) (Herman, 1992; Pelcovitz et al., 1997; van der Kolk, Roth, Pelcovitz, & Mandel, 1993).

2.2   PTSD and Memory

> *Give sorrow words;*
> *The grief that does not speak*
> *Whispers the o'er-fraught heart,*
> *And bids it break*
> William Shakespeare, Macbeth

2.2.1 The Nature of Traumatic Memory

For the development of effective treatment methods, it is essential to understand the psychological and biological processes that underlie disorders of the trauma spectrum including PTSD. Some key features of memories of traumatic events emphasize the relevance of memory processes for the explanation of PTSD symptoms.

The most distinct symptom of PTSD is the reexperiencing of the traumatic event in the form of flashbacks.

These involuntary intrusions can be triggered by cues that remind a person of the traumatic situation. The reliving can include all kinds of sensory information, such as pictures, sounds, smells, and bodily sensations (Terr, 1993; van der Kolk, 1995). A feature of flashbacks is the feeling that this event is happening again right at that very moment. This means that during a flashback, victims are not fully aware that what they are experiencing is active memory arising from past experiences; on the contrary, they think they are back in the traumatic situation. The memory of the traumatic event does not seem to be fixed in the context of the time and space in which it actually occurred (Ehlers & Clark, 2000).

The person may see, feel, or hear the sensory elements of the traumatic experience, yet he or she may be prevented from being able to translate this experience into communicable language. Despite the fact that patients report frequent episodes of reliving the experience through flashbacks or nightmares, it is extremely difficult for them to narrate the event in a detailed consistent and chronological manner. Patients report that they can remember the event all too well, as they suffer from painful involuntary recollections. However, if asked to report the event, the narrations are typically disorganized, fragmented, and incoherent (van der Kolk, 1995). As Herman (1992) puts it, humans who have survived atrocities often tell their stories in a highly emotional, contradictory, and fragmented manner which undermines their credibility and thereby serves the twin imperatives of truth-telling and secrecy. Survivors can begin their recovery only when the truth is finally acknowledged. But "secrecy prevails, and the story of the traumatic event surfaces not as a verbal narrative but as a symptom" (Herman, 1992).

Harvey and Bryant (1999) showed that the disorganization of the narration is correlated with symptoms of acute stress disorder. Systematic observations found evidence that there is a breakdown in the ability to put the most emotional part of the traumatic event, over a period of time which could have lasted anywhere from several seconds to hours or even days, into words. Bessel van der Kolk (1997) has argued that trauma is experienced as "timeless and ego-alien." Victims may literally be out of touch with their feelings. Physiologically, they may respond as if they are being traumatized again, but this may be dissociated from semantic knowledge – not part of the explicit memory. If the victim experiences de-realization he cannot "own" what is happening, and thus cannot take steps to do anything about it.

For survivors of longer-lasting events and for those who were exposed to a series of traumatic events, as is often the case for victims of organized or family violence (especially childhood abuse), this problem in narrating one's history can persist for a long period of time. This effect was described by Rosenthal (1997), who documented the life stories of Holocaust survivors:

> It is difficult to establish a relationship between the different stages of life – this means the time before the persecution, the time of persecution and the time after having survived. Within these stages, the relationship of the different events can be substantially broken into pieces. Whole stages can sink into the sphere of speechlessness and are accessible for the biographer only in single fragments, pictures and moods. (p. 40)

Thus, the characteristic of the memory of a traumatic event is twofold: On the one hand, a person has very vivid recollections of the event including many sensory details; on the other hand, it is very difficult for the victim to face the memories and to learn to put the details into coherent speech and chronological order. This is because traumatic events are stored differently from memories of everyday events. This pathological representation of traumatic memories is what is responsible for the core symptoms of PTSD (Brewin, 2001; Brewin, Dalgleish, & Joseph, 1996; Ehlers & Clark, 2000; Metcalfe & Jacobs, 1996; van der Kolk, 1996). This difference in storage of memories will be addressed next.

To understand the pathological characteristics of traumatic memories, it is first necessary to understand how normal past events are stored in memory. Based on neuropsychological research, Squire (1994) differentiated two types of memory: declarative (explicit) and nondeclarative (implicit). Declarative memory consists of memory of personal events, as well as memory of facts and knowledge of the world. For instance, declarative memory represents significant events such as a marriage or a graduation, as well as knowledge about the history or geography of the world. In contrast, nondeclarative memory covers skills, habits, emotional associations, and conditioned responses. Based on this taxonomy of memory, Squire (1994) determined that declarative or explicit memories can be deliberately retrieved, whereas nondeclarative or implicit memories are not deliberately retrieved and do not require conscious recollection. Nondeclarative memories do have an impact on a person's behavior and experiences, but are activated through other processes, such as environmental or internal cues, similar to the memories of trauma survivors.

Using the example of declarative memory, we know that the memory of a wedding or the story of the French Revolution can be deliberately retrieved or activated when desired (assuming one was paying attention in history class!). However, nondeclarative memories do not involve a deliberate recall. For example, for most people, opening a door is a highly practiced skill that is automatically activated without ever remembering how and when that skill was learned. The memory of a traumatic event can be triggered by an external cue such as a smell or a sound. Putting these two types of memory together, we can see that a single event can be stored as two different types of memory. For instance, a person learns to ride a bike. The day the rider learned to ride the bike is stored in that person's memory as a historical, autobiographical event in that person's life. This is an example of declarative memory. However, as the person becomes more adept at bike riding, it is no longer necessary to remember each step of riding the bike. Riding a bike thus becomes a skill that is easily activated without deliberate recall. It is coded as a nondeclarative memory.

Tulving (2001) further distinguished between *episodic* and *semantic* memory. As the name implies, episodic memories are stored as episodes, i.e., happenings in particular places at particular times, and cover information about what, where, and when. Tied to episodic memory is the recollective experience. Episodic memory allows people to consciously reexperience previous events and to activate their sensory-perceptual experience. In contrast, semantic memory is our knowledge base – for instance, it might include knowing that five times 12 equals 60 or that Greenland is covered with ice. This type of memory is not necessarily related to experience in the sense that a visit to Greenland has to be made to build up the respective semantic representation.

2.2.2 Sensory-Perceptual Representation

If you think about past life events, you may not only retrieve abstract knowledge about what has happened ("On September 21st, I went to Jaffna by boat"), but also sometimes imagine the event in the form of a "recollective experience" (Tulving, 2001) ("I feel the breeze over the water, the swinging of the boat"). In the case of recalling the event as a recollective experience, you directly access visual and other sensory information about past events previously stored in your mind, in addition to being aware of the sequence of events that happened.

Obviously, this form of vivid and detailed recollection is not possible for all events experienced in life.

For everyday events, which have less significance to a person, these representations usually only last minutes or hours (Conway, 2001). They can only become more stable if they are integrated with other memory structures. In this case, detailed images of this event can be retrieved years later. This enduring storage of sensory-perceptual representations only happens for events stored in a highly emotional state, as this means they are significant for the achievement or failure of individual goals (Conway & Pleydell-Pearce, 2000).

Lang's bioinformational theory of emotion (Lang, 1979) offers a good framework within which to understand the nature of sensory-perceptual representations and their embedding emotions. In this view, emotions are considered "response propositions" or more general action dispositions, i.e., modes in neural networks (neuronal connections within the brain) that favor distinct sets of actions.

These representations consist of sensory-perceptual information about the stimuli present in the past situation in different modalities (visual, auditory, olfactory, etc.). In other words, a single traumatic memory can be experienced by a victim in many different ways, all simultaneously. At the same time as a person is experiencing the sensory aspects of the memory, for instance, other parts of this network or system within the brain are processing cognitive or emotional information in response to the stimuli. Additionally, the body is also responding with a set of corresponding physiological reactions. Another set of response propositions include the motor and physiological responses to the stimulus or memory. All elements of this network of brain activity are connected such that the activation of a single item (such as a sensory experience) leads to an activation of other elements (see Figure 4 as an example).

The sensory-perceptual representations of traumatic events have also been called "fear structures." Lang (1979, 1984, 1993) concluded that fear structures or fear networks operate in anxiety disorders. This theory explains the ability to remember and relive past events in the form of "recollective experiences" (in which the subjective, sensory components of memory are experienced; as conceptualized by Tulving (2001)). In addition, this model predicts that these recollections of the event would occur simultaneously with physiological and emotional responses similar to those that occurred when the event happened. For instance, if someone experienced great levels of fear and terror accompanied by heart palpitations while watching a horrible event,

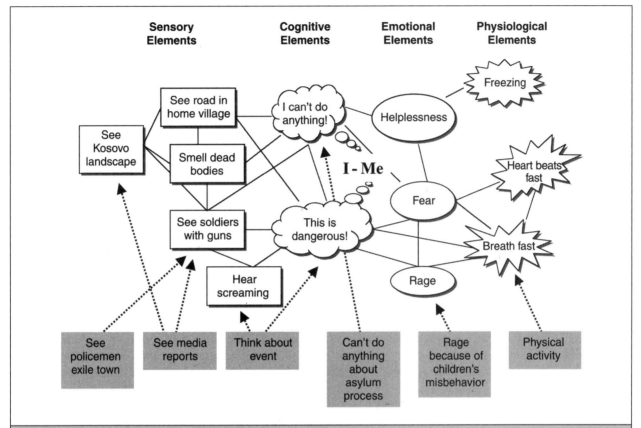

Figure 4. Schematic presentation of a hypothetical sensory-perceptual representation, including sensory, cognitive, emotional, and physiological elements. The network represents a Kosovar refugee's memory of the attack on his home village. The boxes below indicate environmental stimuli with the potential to activate the representation.

this fear and terror and the heart palpitations would be relived upon remembering the event. These predictions have been confirmed by Lang (1979, 1984, 1993) and coworkers using subjective, behavioral, and physiological measurements during mental imagery.

Conway (2001) stated that the retrieval of a sensory-perceptual representation, a memory with sensory information, is the final step in recalling a memory of a past event. He asserts that this process of recovering sensory information takes some effort on the part of the individual and that the process lasts for several seconds of time, rather than occurring instantaneously. However, the impact of emotional structures on behavior is not limited to the deliberate retrieval of memories of past events, as for instance during voluntary mental imagery. Elements of the structure can also be automatically retrieved by a cue, and lead to emotional behavior. For instance, the smell of dead bodies may activate pictures of a road in the home village in the network of Figure 4, without the person choosing to bring these pictures back to mind. Edna Foa and Mike Kozak, a Lang scholar, have related the network theory to PTSD (Foa & Kozak, 1986), whereby a PTSD net-

work would differ from representations (the coding of memories) of normal events in several ways:

- Fear structures encoded during a traumatic event are unusually large (including many nodes or neural elements within the brain) and cover a wide variety of single elements being coded, such as sight, sound, different emotions, and physical sensations. This means that nodes in the fear/trauma structures can be easily activated, as many stimuli in the environment have similarities to one or the other element and thus can act as cues (see also Figure 6).
- Interconnections between single elements, such as sight and sound, are unusually powerful. Consequently, the ignition of only a single element, such as a firecracker exploding, may be sufficient to activate the whole structure, causing all of the related memories to return. This explains why traumatized people can have sudden flashbacks when reminded of the traumatic event. According to this theory, an environmental stimulus or internal cue, such as thinking about the event or an intense heartbeat that resembles one part of the stimulus configuration of the traumatic situation can cause the full firing of the sensory information. In turn, the associat-

ed emotional, physiological, and motor responses stored in the fear/trauma structure will also be triggered. According to this theory, a flashback is the activation of the entire fear/trauma network.

In addition to phenomena of intrusive recollections, this theory can also explain the typical PTSD symptom of avoidance. The activation of a fear structure is experienced as a fearful and painful recollection, and consequently many PTSD patients learn to prevent this by avoiding cues that remind them of the traumatic event. They learn to avoid both internal and external cues, so they try not to think about it, not to talk about it, and to keep away from persons and places that remind them of the event. In addition, running away or other types of motoric flight behavior (feeling the need to flee a specific situation) can be part of the fear/trauma structure. The potential of physiological arousal to trigger the fear network can be so strong that any affective arousal, even positive emotions, are avoided. The victim seems to have become emotionally numb.

2.2.3 Autobiographical Contextual Memory

The sensory-perceptual representation is only one type of memory about past experiences. When a person retrieves a memory about a past event, the type of memory that is generally retrieved first is called "autobiographical memory" (see Figure 5) (Conway & Pleydell-Pearce, 2000). At the top of the hierarchy of autobiographical memory organization is the memory of *lifetime periods*. Lifetime periods represent general knowledge of persons, places, actions, activities, plans, or goals that characterize a special period. They cover distinct time periods with identifiable beginnings and endings. An example of a lifetime period is "the time when I lived with Mary." Lifetime periods are typically organized along major themes of persons who are related to goals in life. Typical themes include relationships, occupations, and places one lived. Lifetime periods related to different themes can overlap with respect to the time period to which they refer. For example, the time covered by "when I was working at the farm" may overlap with the time span of "when I lived with Mary."

A type of knowledge base, or classification of memories, one step down from lifetime periods is the memory of *general events*. General events can be divided into repeated events such as "having lunch at the cafeteria" or single events such as "my first day at school." These knowledge bases organize the sequence of events. Not all events a person experiences are represented with the same accuracy. Shum (1998) suggested that those

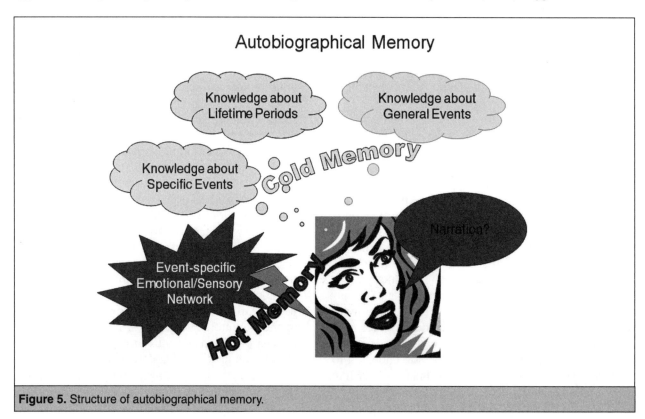

Figure 5. Structure of autobiographical memory.

events demarcating beginnings and ends of lifetime periods play a significant role in defining autobiographical memories. These landmark events (like the first date with a subsequent intimate partner or the struggle that indicated the end of a relationship) are thought to be represented in more detail and accessed more easily. Memories of activities that cover a series of events related to a common theme can be connected to form so-called mini-histories (Robinson, 1992). For example, the mini-history of "my first love" consists of a set of memories of related events such as "my first date" and "my first kiss."

Continuing down the hierarchy of memory, Conway and Pleydell-Pearce (2000) define *event-specific knowledge*. This knowledge corresponds to the sensory-perceptual representations described above, such as "when my mother was taking me to school" (on my first day at school). Event specific knowledge (mother was taking me to school) is usually linked to general event structures ("my first day at school"), and the activation of the sensory-perceptual details of an event (e.g., the picture of the classroom) is accompanied by the activation of knowledge about the sequence of the event ("first we went to school, and then I saw the classroom") and the location of the event in lifetime periods ("we still lived in our homeland then"). As an exercise, the reader may mark the following as either life-time periods, general/specific events, or emotional/sensory network:

I remember this warm day in spring. It was near my parent's house, some 20 years ago. I was still going to kindergarten, it was my last year before primary school. My father had bought me a blue bike the day before. He was pushing me, and I can remember well the exciting feeling I had when I started rolling on my own. I was tense but very happy at the same time! I had the feeling "yes I can!"

Taking this new understanding of memory, we can now look at PTSD and how memory is affected (Figure 6). First, we will take a closer look at how autobiographical memory, general memory, and lifetime periods are all affected in persons with PTSD. The first assumption is that patients who suffer from PTSD have a *significant distortion in their autobiographical memory*. In contrast to those who remember major events as general events, there is evidence to suggest that in persons with PTSD, the traumatic event is *not* clearly represented as a general event. Furthermore, the event does not seem to be clearly positioned in a lifetime period. Even though one's memories and the sensory-perceptual representations of traumatic events are very strong and long lasting, there does not seem to be a reliable auto-

biographical structure within which the memory falls (Figure 6b). Because the ability to recall one's life history in the form of a well-organized autobiographical memory is necessary in order to narrate an event, PTSD patients are often unable to narrate their traumatic experiences. The result is a disorganization and distortion of the sequence of autobiographical memories. In this passage, Metcalfe and Jacobs (1996) describe the typical characteristics of an isolated activation of a sensory-perceptual representation for patients with PTSD:

Memories and reactions that are attributable to the isolated hot-system encoding may seem irrational both to the individual him- or herself, and to the therapist, since such fragments are ungrounded by the kind of narrative and spatio-temporal contextual anchors that tie our ordinary experience to reality. Such memories are disturbing, not only because of the direct fear they evoke, but also because of their strangeness. (p. 2)

The sensory-perceptual-emotional representations of the traumatic event have also been called *hot memory* (Metcalfe & Jacobs, 1996) or *situationally accessible memory*, whereas the autobiographical context memory has been called *cold memory* or *verbally accessible memory*.

Figure 6 illustrates the idea that exposure to different types of severe stressors increases the probability of developing mental health problems: Each stressor incrementally enlarges a neural representational network connected to fear and helplessness. This phenomenon is referred to as the building block effect (Figure 3). Given a high enough level of cumulative exposure to threatening stressors that elicit alarm responses in the mind and body of a survivor, it will eventually wipe out all protective factors that might initially help to counter the onset of a psychiatric illness, notably PTSD and depression. Thereby the brain's networks will integrate experiences of abuse (emotional or physical) and neglect during childhood with those experiences later in life that relate to fear and depression. This may explain the somewhat surprising observation that stressors may make a survivor more vulnerable when they are experienced in quite different contexts rather then the same environment.

Summary PTSD and memory

During a traumatic event, mainly sensory and perceptual information (e.g., the sound of bullet shots or the smell of blood) is stored in memory during a highly emotional state. The mind and body become extremely aroused

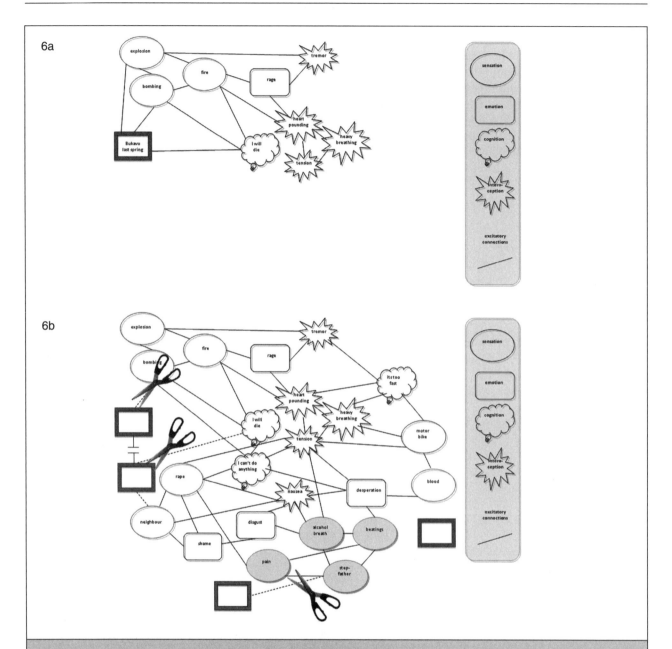

Figure 6. Schematic presentation of a fear/trauma network resulting from multiple traumatic experiences: (a) the experience of a single traumatic event – such as in this case, the experience of a bombing in the city of Bukavu last spring – is well connected to autobiographical memory. (b) If, however, the same experience is integrated into an already existing network of traumatic memories (experiences of domestic violence, earlier accidents, etc.), the connection to the "cold" autobiography gets lost. The sensory, cognitive, emotional, and physiological elements interconnect with increasingly mutual excitatory power. The elements of the cold autobiographical memory, the codes for the where and when, however, inhibit each other, as the brain's architecture does not allow the activation of representations of two different places or two different periods at the same time. The memory for the where – the location, for instance – is coded by "place cells" in the hippocampus. These are neurons that exhibit a high rate of firing whenever the person is actually at the specific location or imagines himself or herself to be in an environment corresponding to the cells' "place field." As only one set of cells can remain active at any given time, the fear/trauma network gets disconnected (symbolized by the scissors) from time and place, and the fear generalizes, giving rise to a permanent feeling of impending threat. Adapted by permission from "Dissociation following traumatic stress: Etiology and treatment" by Maggie Schauer and Thomas Elbert, *Zeitschrift für Psychologie/Journal of Psychology, 218,* 109–127 (doi: 10.1027/0044-3409/a000018). © 2010 Hogrefe Publishing.

(rapid heartbeat, sweating, and trembling) and are set for actions such as hiding, fighting, or running away. This emotional and sensory information is stored separately from the information related to the content. It is stored in an interconnected neural network which may establish a so-called fear network (Figures 4 and 6). This fear/trauma network includes sensory, cognitive, physiological, and emotional experiences, including the action disposition related to the experience (= hot memory, situationally accessible memory, sensory perceptual representation). Environmental stimuli (e.g., a smell or noise) and internal cues (e.g., a thought) can activate this fear/trauma structure later at any given time. The ignition of only a few elements in the network is sufficient to activate the whole structure. This is thought to be a flashback, i.e., the feeling as if one is back in the traumatic situation with its sounds, smells, feelings of fear, response propositions, and thoughts. Since the activation of the fear network is a frightening and painful recollection, many PTSD patients learn to avoid cues that act as reminders of the traumatic event. They try not to think about any part represented in the fear/trauma network, not to talk about it, and to keep away from persons and places that remind them of the frightening event. In contrast to the extensive fear memory, patients who suffer from PTSD have difficulties with autobiographical memory; that is, they are unable to place the fear of the events appropriately in time and space and to clearly position them in a lifetime period (Figure 5). This, and the avoidance of activating the fear/trauma structure, makes it difficult for PTSD patients to narrate their traumatic experience.

2.2.4 Neurobiological Basis of Memory and PTSD

A recognition of how memories are formed and coded within the brain is the next step in understanding the potential impairment that might occur with a person suffering from PTSD. Neuroimaging studies have demonstrated significant neurobiological changes in PTSD. There appear to be several areas of the brain in particular that are different in patients with PTSD compared with those in control subjects: the hippocampus, the amygdala, and the medial prefrontal cortex, which includes the anterior cingulate cortex (Kolassa & Elbert, 2007). The medial temporal lobe and the connected hippocampus are brain structures that play a major role in the transformation and construction of the (cold) memories that contain autobiographical information, including the temporal and spatial context of an event. Thus these neurocircuits are vital to episodic memory formation and emotional regulation by putting specific events into their proper context, binding together multiple events that co-occur during

an experience, and converting short-term into long-term memories: i.e., they play a central role in the encoding of context, also during fear conditioning. McClelland and colleagues (McClelland, McNaughton, & O'Reilly, 1995) suggested that the hippocampus is especially important for the coding of information that contradicts previously learned knowledge. This is especially important for survivors of traumatic experiences, as much of what they experience during times of trauma contradicts basic assumptions that have been learned in life about security, trust, and human nature. The amygdala and cingulate cortex are relevant for *hot* memories. The amygdala is involved in the assessment of threat-related stimuli and has been suggested to be at the center of the defense cascade involved in the acquisition and expression of conditioned fear. It receives information from all sensory modalities and projects to various subcortical structures involved in mediating specific signs of fear and anxiety: e.g., facial expression of fear, stress hormone release, galvanic skin response, blood pressure elevation, hypoalgesia, and freezing. The amygdala thus plays a pivotal role in mediating stress-related effects on behavior and modulating hippocampal function. The medial prefrontal cortex inhibits activation of the amygdala and is involved in the extinction of conditioned fear. It includes the anterior cingulate cortex, which is implicated in evaluating the emotional significance of stimuli and in attentional function (Cardinal, Parkinson, Hall, & Everitt, 2002).

In PTSD, the amygdala appears to be hyperreactive to trauma-related stimuli. In turn, higher brain regions, such as the hippocampus and the medial frontal cortex, are affected, as they are unable to handle the overload of stimuli that results from symptoms such as an exaggerated startle response and flashbacks. Stress hormones that result from these experiences impair the ability of the brain to function properly and to create memories correctly. Based on research with rodents (for a review, see, e.g., McEwen, 2002), there is evidence that the stress hormones released during traumatic events affect both the function and the structure of the hippocampus. Exposure to glucocorticoids (stress hormones that occur during traumatic events) normally increases the activity of the hippocampus; however, if a certain threshold is exceeded, its functioning begins to decline drastically. Under very high levels of stress, the functioning of the hippocampus becomes severely impaired, and the hippocampus, along with the medial frontal cortex, is unable to mediate the exaggerated symptoms of arousal and distress that occur in the amygdala in response to reminders of the traumatic event (Nutt & Malizia, 2004). In animals,

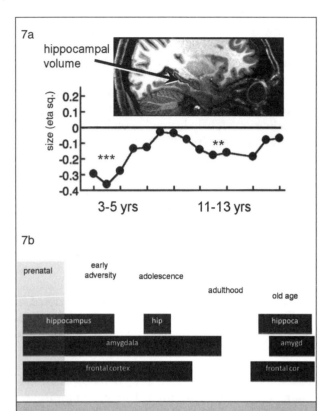

Figure 7. (a) Depending on the developmental period, chronic or repeated exposure to traumatic stressors may significantly reduce (negative values) hippocampal volume later in life (data from Andersen, & Teicher, 2008). (b) The sensitivity of brain regions to alter their structure in response to stressors varies with developmental periods.

very high doses of adrenal steroids may even cause permanent and irreversible atrophy (decrease in size) of the hippocampus (Kim & Yoon, 1998; McEwen, 1999). In humans, a series of cross-sectional studies examined structural abnormalities of the hippocampus and other brain regions in subjects with various traumata. Originally, Bremner et al. (1997, 2003) reported that the hippocampus is smaller in individuals with PTSD than in comparison subjects. Subsequently, it became increasingly evident that this effect of a sizeable volumetric reduction depends on the developmental period when the traumatic stress has been experienced first (see Figure 7). When drug intake, such as excessive alcohol consumption, is controlled, traumatic stress in adults, even when severe, such as in torture survivors, will not result in a reduction of hippocampal volume (Eckart et al., 2010). With respect to functional changes, the findings are mixed, ranging from no or lower activation of the hippocampus during cognitive tasks, to increased hippocampal activation when at rest or across tasks (cf. Shin, Rauch, & Pitman, 2006).

Several studies found changes in the limbic cortex, and particularly in the anterior cingulate cortex. Some authors have argued that the cause–effect relationship is preexisting – i.e., that an individual with a smaller hippocampus may be more prone to develop PTSD when exposed to a traumatic event – and these researchers explored whether or not a reduction in the volume of the hippocampus occurs in survivors of a recent trauma who develop PTSD. Shalev and his group found that smaller hippocampal volume is not a preexisting risk factor for the development of PTSD, but that it later occurs in individuals with chronic or complicated PTSD (Bonne et al., 2001).

In our own research, we have identified structural alterations of the cortex (Eckart et al., 2010): PTSD patients (and to a lesser extent, trauma-exposed controls) showed reduced gray matter volumes in the right inferior parietal cortex, the left rostral middle frontal cortex, the bilateral lateral orbitofrontal cortex, and the bilateral isthmus of the cingulate. An influence of cumulative exposure to traumatic stress on the isthmus of the cingulate and the lateral orbitofrontal cortex indicated that, at least in these regions, structural alterations might be associated with repeated stress experience. These results indicate that lateral prefrontal, parietal, and posterior midline structures become structurally remodeled by repeated traumatic stress experiences. As these regions are particularly involved in episodic memory, emotional processing, and executive control, these changes might be part of the physiological substrate of PTSD symptoms. In addition to these massive structural changes, there are other brain regions that show functional alterations in survivors of

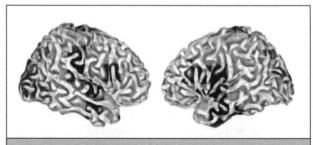

Figure 8. Abnormal brain waves have been recorded and localized in brains of a torture victim, using magnetic source imaging. Volume elements (voxels) where abnormal brain waves are generated have been marked with darker shades of gray. Examples of abnormal oscillatory activity as shown here include frontotemporal regions, notably the insula and the region around Broca's area in the left hemisphere. Abnormality in these regions may be related to the "speechlessness" of the terror. (Data from our clinic, see also Kolassa et al., 2007).

organized violence: We observed massively changed oscillatory properties in left temporal brain regions, with peak activities in the region of the insula (Figure 8). Furthermore, we found altered slow wave activity in right frontal areas in PTSD patients compared with controls (Kolassa et al., 2007). The insula, as a site of multimodal convergence, could play a key role in understanding central aspects of PTSD, possibly accounting for what has been called posttraumatic alexithymia, i.e., a reduced ability to identify, express, and regulate emotional responses to reminders of traumatic events. Differences in activity in right frontal areas may indicate a dysfunctional prefrontal cortex, which may lead to diminished extinction of conditioned fear and reduced inhibition of the amygdala.

Summary   PTSD and the brain

The functioning of brain structures important for memory coding, such as the medial temporal lobe including the hippocampus, is strongly affected by traumatic stress via stress hormones. Under very high levels of traumatic stress, the function of the hippocampus and related neural networks becomes impaired. The fear/trauma network, at first activates multiple but incompatible sets of place cells. Their parallel activation produces mainly noise in the hippocampus. During times of severe stress, this adds to the distorted autobiographical memory storage. Other brain areas are affected in turn (inferior parietal cortex, middle frontal cortex, lateral orbitofrontal cortex, and the isthmus of the cingulate, which is an important connection to the hippocampus). On the other hand, the more difficult a stressor is emotionally, the more active those areas of the brain become which encode emotional content, such as the amygdala – the structure in the brain that prepares the body for danger. During a traumatic event and later in response to a reminder of the trauma, the amygdala and the interconnected frontal lobe regions respond ever more vigorously to the stimuli of the event. The individual then is "over-conditioned" to respond to fear. This may explain the exaggerated emotional responses to fear situations in PTSD patients.

2.3   Processing of Affective Experiences

2.3.1 Normal Emotional Processing

Whereas most people react with intensive emotional upheaval or a massive dissociative response immediately following a traumatic event – including symptoms of acute stress and PTSD symptoms – only a minority of this population fully develops chronic PTSD.

Recovery from acute stress symptoms seems to be the usual process in human beings who have been exposed to isolated events. Several authors have tried to identify the mechanisms behind this emotional processing, as this information may lead to the development of effective treatment options for chronic PTSD. In an influential work on the topic, Foa and Kozak (1986) suggested that *emotional processing* involves a modification of the original fear/trauma structure; in other words, the fear/trauma structure, or the complete process of cognitive, psychological, and physiological events that occur when a person is remembering a fearful event, is modified such that the complete fear/trauma structure is no longer triggered by current events and stimuli (see Section 2.2.2 for a discussion of fear/trauma structures).

In order for the victim to recover from the debilitating effects of PTSD, the mind and brain must begin to *control or inhibit the fear response,* leading to a modification or extinction of the fear/trauma network. One theory is that by activating the fear/trauma structure in a safe context, for example, by allowing the memories to be triggered with another person present, this process can begin to take place. Triggering the memories in a momentarily safe environment allows for the possibility of introducing new elements, ones that are incompatible with the original fear-based connections, into the existing fear/trauma structure. For example, the newly introduced thought or cognition "I am safe" contradicts the main cognitive elements of the fear structure that have been resulting in a permanent state of impending threat. By allowing the individual to experience the current fear structure in conjunction with the current incompatible information, the fear structure can be modified such that maladaptive associations between the stimulus (fearful memories) and response (symptoms of PTSD) decrease over time. In other words, by exposing the individual to both the triggers to the fearful memories of the trauma, along with new contradictory information, the fear will begin to lessen over time as the new information is integrated. Normally, this process of integration occurs naturally after an emotional event without any specific intervention, but in the case of extreme traumatic stress, it may be inhibited due to an avoidance of the fear/trauma structure or because the individual prematurely terminates the process out of fear of the stimuli. Moreover, repeated stress will enlarge and reinforce the fear/trauma structure while disconnecting its elements from the contextual cues (when and where the traumatic stressor has been experienced) at the same time. This will lead to the development of chronic PTSD.

Research on *fear conditioning* has challenged this view. Several investigators have shown that an *extinction or elimination of fear responses* will not necessarily change the original stimulus–fear associations, as the original fear response can easily be reinstated in a context different from the context of extinction learning. For example, just because an individual has become accustomed or desensitized to hearing fireworks does not mean that a repeated traumatic event will not reinstate the original fear structure. Instead, extinction probably occurs through the inhibition of the fear response by a *regulative process* (LeDoux, 2000). This regulative process is based on a more thorough evaluation of the current situation than the automatic evaluation by the fear structure – that is, the brain is able to process the information about the event more slowly and thoroughly rather than just reacting emotionally to the information. Brewin (2001) suggested that this cortical evaluation depends on the availability of declarative memory of the stimulus. By using the information from declarative memory about the past event, the individual is better able to evaluate whether the current stimulus indicates a threat.

As noted above, after a traumatic event, declarative knowledge, and especially autobiographical knowledge, which offers information about the context of the feared stimulus, is fragmented or even absent. This can lead to a lack of capability for the *cortical inhibitory control of the fear response*. The process of cortical inhibition of the conditioned fear response occurs as the person learns to distinguish between past and present threats. In other words, the person who experienced a traumatic event in the past learns that stimuli in the present are not currently a threat. In normal emotional processing, the intrusive memories provide an opportunity for the individual to build up declarative memory about the event. As the person thinks and talks about this event, utilizing and integrating the memories and the stimuli presented by intrusive memories, cortical regulation begins to take place, and more functional and accurate autobiographical knowledge

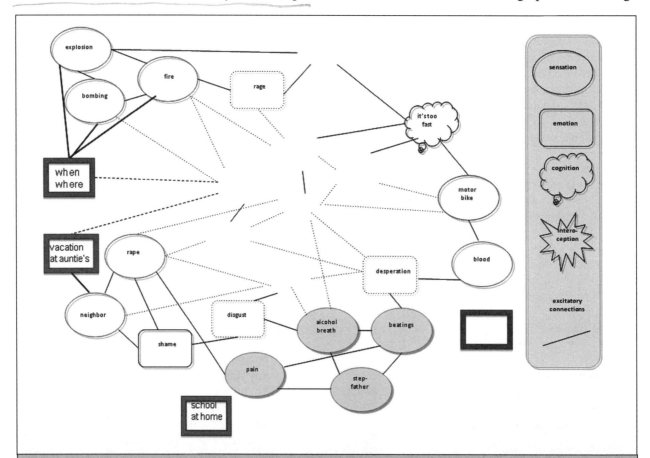

Figure 9. Connecting the cold, declarative elements to the hot memories will fractionize the fear/trauma network into its original elements. Cues are less likely to trigger neural representations of all the traumatic memories, but will activate a subset of representations, related to a particular traumatic event. The survivor will realize that the activated cognitions, emotions, and sensory elements relate to the past and no longer to the present.

can be constructed about the traumatic episode. The construction of autobiographical knowledge about the traumatic event is no easy task, as the organization of autobiographical knowledge is connected to personal goals and to basic beliefs about the self. This means that active emotional processing takes time and effort. Secondary emotions such as anger and guilt may indicate problems in the cognitive processing of the event and the adaptive placement of the traumatic experience in the context of preexisting beliefs about the self, which also interferes with the construction of a coherent autobiographical representation. Because thinking about the traumatic event automatically causes painful emotions, many people avoid this process and try to eliminate intrusive memories as soon as possible. The fact that victims with poor social support following a traumatic event are at an increased risk for developing PTSD (Ozer, Best, Lipsey, & Weiss, 2003) might be explained by the lack of opportunity or encouragement to talk about the event. Persons who do not have strong support networks may be less likely to talk about the event, which would allow for emotional processing and the chronological reconstruction of autobiographical memory.

Summary	Emotional processing of the fear/trauma structure

Emotional processing enables the reconstruction of the autobiographical representation of the event. The explicit (declarative) autobiographical representation is needed to regulate the activation of the original fear/trauma structure. This will modify the connections within the fear/trauma structure (Figure 9). People naturally seem to try to heal themselves by narrating their experiences. In many cases this is helpful, because this process naturally helps building up cool memory context information. Because thinking about the traumatic event automatically causes painful emotions, people avoid this process (despite the fact that it may prove helpful) and try to terminate recollection as soon as possible. By avoiding the memories, they are inhibiting the habitual processing of the experience, and as a result the fear/trauma structure seems to consolidate itself, and chronic PTSD can develop. When, however, a patient thinks and talks about the event in chronological order and includes the stimuli presented by intrusive memories, autobiographical knowledge about the traumatic episode can be reconstructed, and the victim can learn to distinguish between past and current threats. The construction of a narration enforces the activation and consequently the habituation of the fear. This exposure is the most powerful means to tearing down the fear/trauma network. In this process, the patient is learning that sensory and emotional memory can be activated without fear.

2.3.2 Implications for Treatment

Quite a number of treatment approaches intend to relieve trauma symptoms by purposefully visualizing the traumatic events. Some successfully reduce symptoms having the survivor tell the worst event repeatedly in detail (Bisbey & Bisbey, 1998). Foa and colleagues (Foa & Rothbaum, 1998) systematically developed *exposure therapy* for PTSD. This technique has proven to be one of the most successful treatment approaches for this disorder (Foa et al., 1999). When implementing exposure therapy for PTSD, the patient is instructed to repeatedly talk about the traumatic experience, thus exposing the individual to the event and memories. Likewise controlled, randomized studies have shown the superiority of exposure elements in cognitive behavior treatment in children and adolescents compared to other approaches (Saigh, 1992; Saigh, Yule, & Inamdar, 1996). In particular, Foa (Foa et al., 1995) demonstrated that those patients who manage to construct a coherent narrative of the event during exposure therapy profit most from treatment.

The main focus of this therapy should be on the part of the memory that is most fragmented in autobiography and most intensively represented in sensory-perceptual representations. These moments of intense recollection of memories, complete with physical sensations, have often been referred to as "hot spots." In order for the victim to form a consistent autobiographical narration of this moment, the *sensory-perceptual representations (memories of physical sensations)* are inevitably activated, as they provide detailed knowledge about the event that is not yet available in *declarative (autobiographical) structures*. When recovering or recreating the autobiographical memories of the event, the patient should be encouraged to relay those memories that have the highest probability of eliciting intrusive symptoms, such as flashbacks or physical sensations. Because the sensory-perceptual representations of the memories in the brain provoke intense emotional reactions, successful therapy cannot proceed without a high level of emotional involvement.

Consistent with this view, Jaycox, Foa, and Morral (1998) showed that treatment success in exposure therapy is positively correlated with the level of fear initially experienced in treatment – that is, the higher the level of fear experienced initially, the greater the success of the treatment. The task of a therapist is therefore to encourage the activation of painful memories and to prevent the patient's habitual strategies of avoiding or ending the activation. At the same time, the therapist should assist the patient in organizing the declarative or autobiographical memories related to the traumatic event and in placing the event in time and space (Figure 9). *Habituation* of the emotional response occurs as the memories are no longer capable of eliciting the response part of the fear network. As habituation takes place, the telling of the memories will no longer evoke strong emotional reactions, confusion, and fear in the patient.

Associations between stimuli and fear responses cannot always be erased in therapy of PTSD patients. For certain individuals, there may always be some fear that is evoked upon remembering the event. Instead of attempting to extinguish all fear through habituation, new associations with the stimuli may need to be established. In this case, the new association would be the declarative or factual knowledge that is constructed and tied to the stimuli that provoke intrusive symptoms. For instance, a goal for a victim whose fear is activated by the sight of fire might be to associate some declarative knowledge with the sight of fire, such as the time of day or time of year, rather than the emotional content of the memory. Several repetitions of the new associations may be necessary before the declarative knowledge is the preferred representation that gets activated when reminded of the event. Only after these associations are firmly established will the fear responses and the associated intrusive symptoms be inhibited by the new knowledge base, and a modification of the fear structure initiated.

Note that putting feeling into words regulates negative emotional responses. Linguistic processing such as affect-labeling and naming of emotions control amygdala activity (Hariri, Bookheimer, & Mazziotta, 2000; Lieberman, Hariri, Jarcho, Eisenberger, & Bookheimer, 2005). Affect-labeling, not just the recognition of the emotion as such, disrupts the affective responses and diminishes activity in the limbic system that would otherwise occur in the presence of negative experiences, a process that may ultimately contribute to better mental and physical health (Lieberman, et al. 2007). Throughout the narrative exposure process, the therapist helps the verbalizing, labeling, and clarifying and integrating of emotional responding.

2.3.3 Speechlessness of Trauma: Sociopolitical Implications

In addition to the known fact that psychological trauma is a consequence or outcome of violence, there is also increasing discussion as to whether this psychological trauma can contribute to the number of violent conflicts – family or state violence – in the world. Orga-

nizations that provide psychosocial interventions in war-affected societies have justified their interventions not only as a means of improving mental health care for individuals, but also by making the case that these interventions are relevant to society and on a political scale. One common assertion is that the treatment of so-called traumatized societies is necessary to break the *cycle of trauma and violence* (Tauber, 2003; UNICEF, 2001). The cycle-of-trauma argument implies that victims of violence are more likely to become perpetrators later on. At the same time, treatment of traumatized survivors is considered to facilitate forgivingness and reconciliation within the society.

Whereas it is unclear to what extent and how, political processes affect the mental health of victims, it is very likely that the psychological status of victims has an effect on social and political processes beyond the assumed cycle of trauma. In every society there are individuals who want to speak out about what has happened and to pass their experiences on to their children as well as to the public. Some of them will be able to do so on their own, and many local human rights groups have evolved to give these people a forum. Many survivors of the Holocaust, for example, have chosen to document their own experiences as a means of educating subsequent generations (Bettelheim, 1986; Frankl, 1946).

A considerable number of people, especially those who suffer from PTSD, are unable to narrate their personal histories because of the pathological effects of the traumatic events on their memory. This puts the victims at a disadvantage in comparison with the perpetrators and bystanders, who usually have no difficulties explaining their position. Offering victims a means of processing their traumatic events and documenting their history can help to give them a voice within their society. During the Pinochet regime in Chile, Lira and Weinstein (published under the pseudonyms Cienfuegos & Monelli, 1983) developed *testimony therapy* as a specialized treatment approach for torture victims, which directly addressed this issue.

Testimony therapy is an innovative approach that combines political as well as psychological goals. The biography of the survivor of human rights violations is documented in detail with an emphasis on the persecution history and traumatic events experienced. The resulting documents have been used to accuse the regime of human rights violations and, as a whole, have become a powerful tool in the resistance to the Pinochet dictatorship. Thus, this treatment approach serves two distinct purposes: On the one hand, it serves as a method for facilitating the emotional processing of the victim's traumatic event, resulting in improved mental health, and, at the same time, it acts as a document which can be directly used for political purposes. Other therapists have followed this example and used testimony therapy for different groups of survivors of wars and torture (Agger, 1994; Agger & Jensen, 1990; Weine et al., 1995; Weine & Laub, 1995; Weine, Kulenovic, Pavkovic, & Gibbons, 1998). Despite these reports offering promising results for treatment, testimony therapy has not been widely used in mainstream psychosocial organizations, which primarily favor nonpolitical approaches, such as supportive counseling.

Summary   Treatment of PTSD

Utilizing the memory theory of PTSD, the main goal of therapy is to construct a consistent declarative (autobiographical) representation of the sequence of events experienced by the patient. The act of creating this coherent narrative enables the patient to be exposed to a sensory image of single events (Figure 9). This process allows for habituation and reduces fear responses over time. The task of a therapist is to encourage the activation of painful memories and to prevent the patient's learned strategies of avoiding or ending the activation of these memories and physical sensations. At the same time, the therapist should assist the patient in reorganizing the memories related to the traumatic event and in allowing the patient to place the events in time and space. The visualizing or imagining of the events is necessary for the patient to reconstruct his or her life story and will stimulate the learning that these active neural representations are memories and a not life-threatening presence. The patient will habituate in the process and will become accustomed to remembering the events without activating strong emotional responses.

2.4   Narrative Exposure Therapy (NET): The Theoretical Model

2.4.1   Rationale of NET

Raw experience + meaning = narrative
J. Holmes, in Healing Stories:
Narrative in Psychiatry and Psychotherapy
(Holmes, 1999)

The majority of survivors of organized violence, of war and torture, are unable to safely escape their countries, forced instead to flee to insecure places within their home country or in adjacent regions that are often equally affected by war and terror. In addition to living with violence, many of these refugees are also living in poverty, suffering from malnourishment, and are dependent on humanitarian aid. It seems plausible that these living conditions would question the applicability of any psychotherapeutic treatment. However, experience shows that this is not the case. Contrary to Maslow's hierarchy of needs, suggesting that treatment for psychological problems cannot be addressed as long as the basic needs of nutrition and safety are pressing, our investigations show that survivors see their mental health as having the highest priority and that mental functioning is the prerequisite for self-efficacy and meeting one's basic needs.

The same is often true for survivors of family violence or continuous civil trauma. They are often helpless for many years, if not decades. They experience severe abuse in their homes, and at the same time, they are often isolated and bullied by peers. They often do not have access to help and treatment since they are silenced by the perpetrators and held under threat. Furthermore, the victims' own guilt and feelings of shame hinder their seeking help.

It is true for both survivor groups – those who have suffered complex civil trauma and organized violence – that they have difficulties with mental and daily functioning, which constitute a part of any clinical diagnosis. In turn this hinders autarkic living (economic self-sufficiency) in these persons, as well as social and economic reconstruction and development. Healing of PTSD thus empowers survivors to live self-determined lives. Neither are both groups living in safety, as is often required as a precondition for treatment.

In addition, given the large numbers of people and limited monetary resources in refugee camps and settlements, any psychotherapeutic intervention must be limited in time. Broad-scale treatment programs must be pragmatic and easy for local personnel to learn, even with little or no access to medical or psychological education or additional training. Consequently, the method must be adaptable to multiple cultural environments and easily implemented. The oral tradition is a common element among many cultures; thus narrative approaches, such as NET, seem ideally suited to cross-cultural applications.

NET is an intervention we have developed for the treatment of PTSD resulting from exposure to multiple and continuous traumatic stressors. NET is based on the theory of the fear/trauma network (as outlined in Section 2.2.3) and includes principles of cognitive behavioral exposure therapy and testimony therapy (Neuner et al., 2002, 2004b). In exposure therapy, the patient is requested to repeatedly recall and talk about a traumatic experience in detail while reexperiencing all emotions, bodily sensations, and implicit memory parts associated with this event – but this time emphasizing the time and place of the event. In the process, NET weaves *hot implicit memories* into the story unfolded by *cool declarative memories,* allowing the majority of patients to undergo habituation of the emotional response to the traumatic memory, which consequently leads to a remission of the anxiety disorder. While working through the biography of a person, many positive memories are revisited. Their importance can sink in, and they can become valuable resources for life.

Pure exposure methods usually work with the worst event – i.e., the one traumatic event a person has experienced, assuming that this will lead to the best treatment outcome. However, victims of organized violence, war, and torture have experienced several, often many, traumatic events, and it is often impossible to identify the worst event. NET relies on the chronicity of life: Instead of defining a single event as a target in therapy, patients construct a narration of their whole lives, following the timeline of their lives from birth to the present, while focusing on detailed reports of the traumatic experiences.

Summary   Basic Principles of NET

Narrative exposure therapy (NET) is a treatment approach that was developed for the treatment of PTSD resulting from organized or family violence – multiple and/or continuous trauma(tic) stress(ors). In NET, the patient repeatedly talks about each traumatic event in detail while reexperiencing the emotions, cognitions, physiology, behavioral, and sensory elements and meaning content associated with this event. As well, the patient narrates positive life experiences. With the guiding and directive help of the therapist, the patient constructs a narration of his or her life, focusing on the detailed context of the traumatic experiences as well as on the important elements of the emotional networks and how they go together. This process allows the majority of persons to recognize that the fear/trauma structure results from past experiences and that its activation is nothing but a memory. They thus lose the emotional response to the recollection of the traumatic events, which consequently leads to a remission of PTSD symptoms. At the same time, they gain access to "lost" past memories and develop a sense of coherence, control, and integration.

2.4.2 Elements of NET

The focus of NET is twofold. As with exposure therapy, one goal is to reduce the symptoms of PTSD by confronting the patient with memories of the traumatic event. However, recent theories of PTSD and emotional processing suggest that habituation of the emotional responses is only one of the mechanisms that improve symptoms. Other theories suggest that the distortion of the explicit autobiographical memory of traumatic events leads to a fragmented or inconsistent telling of the narrative of traumatic memories (Ehlers & Clark, 2000). Thus, a second element, the reconstruction of autobiographical memory and a consistent narrative, also should be used in conjunction with exposure therapy.

a) As a prerequisite for the induction of emotional processing, memory traces are reactivated, and the whole fear/trauma structure gets engaged:

b) Emotional episodes are coded in memory as networks of mutually activating information units. According to Lang, when processing the network, activity in one unit is transmitted to adjacent units, and depending on the strength of activation, the entire structure may be engaged (Lang, 1977, 1993).

c) Reactivating consolidated memories makes them sensitive to change (Nader, Schafe, & LeDoux, 2000). Experience in the use of NET with patients has led us to the assumption that patients are not always able to estimate the degree to which the hot memories are problematic in an individual's life or even the content that is encapsulated in these hot memories, especially when the memories are being remembered or recreated outside the context of the whole life story. However, patients may be able to identify these same elements when presented with the task of facing the memories within the context of an autobiographical exploration. Dori Laub and his group at the Archive for Holocaust Testimonies at Yale University reported the following experience with a group of Holocaust survivors. In 1979, a grassroots organization, the Holocaust Survivors Film Project, began videotaping Holocaust survivors and witnesses in New Haven, CT. In 1981, the original collection of testimonies was deposited at Yale University, and the Video Archive for Holocaust Testimonies opened its doors to the public the following year. Since then, the archive has worked to record, collect, and preserve Holocaust witness testimonies, and to make its collection available to researchers, educators, and the general public (http://www.library.yale.edu/testimonies/index.html).

When the first testimony began, everything fell into place, because the power of the testimony silenced all differences. Everyone in the room was transported to another time and place, a setting that had been waiting untouched and unchanged for many years behind locked doors. No one, including the witnesses themselves, knew beforehand what the testimonies would contain; experiences and reflections came out from recesses of memory that the witnesses did not even know they had.

Dori Laub, Fortunoff Video Archive
for Holocaust Testimonies at Yale University

People with PTSD often fail to integrate traumatic experiences into the narrative of their lives. As said before, the survivor often cannot report the related experience in a consistent, chronological order, and thus this person has no explicit link between the various events, life experiences, and the context within which the events occurred. Survivors of continuous trauma often "loose" (i.e., no longer possess) their biography as a whole. Not only are the threats and lifetime periods of horror and suffering not accessible, but the other memories cease to exist alongside. By using NET, we are able to carefully step forward through the complete biography of our patients' lives in chronological order. In telling the story, the patient is exposed to the sensory information that accompanies the memory and to the image of the events themselves. The patient actually engages in his or her own fear/trauma network by narrating the fragments throughout the course of therapy, and he or she is able to reweave the events back into a *cool-system framework* controlling the triggers present with the hot memories. As a result, the accompanying anxiety, which evolved from the strangeness of dissociative fragments, is defused. All somatosensory percepts (physical sensations), cognitions (thoughts), and emotions relevant to the fear/trauma network and involved in the traumatic sequences of memory are comprehensively uncovered in detail as the narrative unfolds. The course of events is established (in time and place), labeled, and transferred into speech until a meaningful and consistent narrative is reached. All traumatic events are revisited until their negative, confusing, horrifying impact dissolves.

Note that the effectiveness of narrative procedures can be explained by the construction of an explicit, semantic representation of the events, coupled with a defractionation of the fear/trauma network and by habituation and inhibition of fear and helplessness. As pointed out by Kaminer (2006) in her literature review, three additional factors may also contribute: (1) emotional catharsis, (2) developing an explanation of the traumatic incidence, and (3) identification of the causes of, and responsibilities for, the horror.

Indeed, these factors are an integral part of NET. Experimental evidence, however, is limited regarding whether in the sense of posttraumatic growth, the traumatic experiences will eventually be seen as the individual's own history of resistance, survival, and thus future resilience. What we know today is that *catharsis* as solely abreaction (in the sense of "letting off steam" through the expression or the reactivation of previously suppressed trauma-related feelings) is not enough as a cure for trauma symptoms. This view mixes cause and effect: Only when this activation of hot memories is closely tied to the cold, explicit representations of the where (place) and when (time) is a healing process initiated. Expressing a high level of affect is a misconceived catharsis and will not lead to clinical improvement if it is not related to cognitive processing (Pennebaker & Seagal, 1999). However, the first deliberate activation of essential parts of the fear/trauma network will necessarily produce strong feelings that become manifest in emotionally arousing expressions which then have to be labeled and integrated. Finally, we should note that the effectiveness of NET does not only rely on the trauma focus, but also on continuous psychoeducation about the men-

Summary Elements of NET
What are the therapeutic elements of NET that have proven effective in trauma treatment? 1. Active chronological reconstruction of the autobiographical/episodic memory. 2. Prolonged exposure to the "hot spots" and full activation of the fear memory to modify the emotional network (i.e., learning to separate the traumatic memory from the conditioned emotional response, and understanding triggers as cues, which are just temporarily associated) through detailed narration and imagination of the traumatic event. 3. Meaningful linkage and integration of physiological, sensory, cognitive, and emotional responses to one's time, space, and life context (i.e., comprehension of the original context of acquisition and the reemergence of the conditioned responses in later life). 4. Cognitive reevaluation of behavior and patterns (i.e., cognitive distortions, automatic thoughts, beliefs, and responses), as well as reinterpretation of the meaning content through reprocessing of negative, fearful, and traumatic events – completion and closure. 5. Revisiting of positive life experiences for (mental) support and to adjust basic assumptions. 6. Regaining of one's dignity through satisfaction of the need for acknowledgment through the explicit human rights orientation of "testifying."

tal suffering, on the restructuring or sometimes even building of context and cold memory, on the "put into words," the linguistic representation of the whole narration and on a subsequent new appraisal of shame, guilt, and the acknowledgment of the events and the suffering by the therapist.

3 The Therapeutic Approach of Narrative Exposure Therapy (NET)

3.1 The Basic Procedure of NET

Within a relatively small number of 90–120-minute sessions, usually about 10, the patient constructs a detailed and consistent narration of his or her biography in cooperation with the therapist. The focus of narrative exposure therapy (NET) lies on the completion and integration of the initial fragments of the traumatic events into a whole, including the sensory, physiological, emotional, and cognitive experiences of the incident. The testimony is written down and, depending on the willingness of the patient, used for documentary purposes later. This procedure has been adapted to the special demands of survivors of violence, such as refugees or victims of familial violence and has evolved to the following standard:

The first step is to conduct an assessment of the individual's mental health status, including a diagnostic evaluation of posttraumatic stress disorder (PTSD). Following this evaluation, a psychoeducational introduction is presented to the survivor, focusing on the explanation of his or her disturbance and symptoms, as well as a statement about the universality of human rights. This is followed by a preparatory introduction to the therapeutic approach. Treatment starts immediately following the initial diagnostic assessment, which also includes collecting demographic data, completing a medical and psychiatric history, and assessing for current complaints.

During a classical treatment of anxiety disorders, the patient is gradually exposed to a hierarchy of increasingly anxiety-provoking stimuli. Correspondingly, it has been suggested to rank the traumatic events according to the extent of the client's avoidance at the beginning of the treatment.

Complex psychological traumata leading to complex traumatic stress disorders result from exposure to severe stressors that are repetitive and/or prolonged, involve harm or abandonment by caregivers, and occur at developmentally vulnerable times in the victim's life (Courtois & Ford, 2009). In the case of complex trauma with its multiple and continuous traumatic experiences, the challenge for the survivor to rank countless single events and compare different types of horror is not only formidable, we think it is inhumane to ask for such decisions. The same is true for survivors of multiple traumatic events including witnessing experiences: Is it worse when the husband was shot, or when the daughter was raped, or was my own being tortured the worst experience in life? Sure, one could ask which memories are more fear-provoking – e.g., when my father broke my leg while abusing me sexually, or when he sold me in that cellar to men filming with a camera, while I was abused? However, each and every one of these horrible traumatic experiences is part of an integral fear network which will be triggered by the any of the respective cues. Not before, but only after the treatment will the patient be able to segregate the stressors and sort the events. In NET there is no need for a hierarchical approach, since we work through and narrate the life of a person in chronological order.

A typical narrative extends over the following topics: Personal background and individual history prior to the first traumatic event;

- Experiences from the beginning of the threat to the first terrifying event;
- Terrifying events;
- History of escape from or ending of violent conditions;
- Life thereafter;
- Plans, hopes, and fears concerning the future.

The psychotherapeutic work, before the first traumatic event on the lifeline is touched, may be used as the time during which a foundation for the process is laid and a good rapport between therapist and patient is established. This time also serves as a tutorial for both therapist and patient. In the beginning it is very important that the patient and therapist feel comfortable communicating with each other, so that the patient understands what is actually expected from him or her in terms of how the process of telling the life events will proceed. Also, during this time, the therapist is able to become familiar with the individual expressions and unique characteristics of the patient. In this warm-up phase, for example, the telling of emotional, warm, or exciting moments in the patient's early life offers itself as a training ground of sorts for emotional processing and communication between patient and therapist.

During the telling of the events in the following phases, the therapist structures the topics and helps to clarify ambiguous descriptions. *The therapist assumes an empathic and accepting role.* Inconsistencies in the patient's report are gently pointed out and often resolved by raising in-depth awareness about recurring bodily sensations or thoughts. The patient is encouraged to describe the traumatic events in as much detail as possible and to reveal the emotions and perceptions experienced at the moment of the retelling as well as at the moment of the traumatic event. The patient is assured that he or she is in full control of the procedure at all times and will not be asked to do anything against his or her will. A translator, oriented beforehand to the psychological goals, may be necessary.

During the session, the therapist writes down a short version of the patient's narration. In the subsequent session, this report is read to the patient, and the patient is asked to correct it and to add details that may have been missed and that he or she feels are very important. Then the next stones and flowers are processed – i.e., additional traumatic experiences are added to the narration. The procedure is repeated in subsequent sessions until a final version of the patient's complete biography is created.

In the last session, this document is read again out loud to the patient. The patient, the translator, if present, and the therapist sign the written narration. One copy of the signed document is handed to the patient; another may be kept for scientific purposes, if needed. With the agreement or request of the patient, another copy may be passed on to human rights organizations as documentation of these events. The document may be used for advocacy purposes or published in some other way, if it can be assured that no harm will result for the patient.

A general guideline for the organization of sessions can be outlined as follows:

Session 1: Diagnosis and psychoeducation.

Session 2: Lifeline.

Session 3: Start of the narration beginning at birth and continuing through to the first traumatic event.

Session 4 and subsequent sessions: Rereading of the narrative collected in previous sessions. Continuing the narration of subsequent life and traumatic events.

Final session: Rereading and signing of the whole document.

Summary   Basic elements of NET

A. Construction of a consistent narrative of the patient's biography.

B. The therapist supports the mental reliving of the events that the patient will go through and the emotional processing that goes along with this. The therapist assists the patient in creating a chronological structure of the initial fragments, emphasizing the time and place, and the traumatic experiences had happened. The therapist assumes an empathic and accepting stance.

C. The therapist writes down the survivor's testimony. In a subsequent session, the material is read to the patient, who is then asked to correct it or add missing details. The procedure is repeated across sessions until a final version of the patient's biography that includes all essential traumatic experiences is reached.

D. In the last session, the survivor, the translator, and the therapist sign the written testimony.

E. The survivor keeps the narrative of his life story. As an eyewitness report, it may serve as documentary evidence for human rights violations or for legal purposes.

3.2   The NET Process Step by Step

3.2.1   Organization of Sessions

NET is a short-term treatment approach that has been tested with varying lengths of treatment. The number of sessions required depends on the setting and the severity of PTSD in your patient. Experiences implementing NET in African refugee settlements indicated that the minimum number of sessions required is four, each about 120 minutes in length. For the treatment of survivors of torture, more sessions (typically 8 to 12, of 90 minutes each) may be necessary. For complex trauma, including comorbid disorders such as borderline personality disorders, even twice this number of sessions maybe required. Ideally, the number of NET sessions should be determined before treatment. This is useful because an open-ended length of treatment may lead to an increase in avoidance. The patient inevitably may avoid discussing the most difficult situations and may prolong recovery and pain indefinitely. On the other hand, if the patient knows that chances to recollect his or her story are limited, the process avoidance will be overcome more easily and the period of suffering, including the duration of fear (of the session that enters the major hotspot) is limited.

Many patients with PTSD also suffer from comorbid disorders (depression, other anxiety disorders). These associated disorders sometimes, but not always, disappear with NET treatment. Then, an extended treatment that includes other specialized cognitive behavioral techniques might be necessary after the NET module. In these cases, we recommend starting with the NET, because many comorbid symptoms can be the consequence of trauma and PTSD and thus already be modified through NET.

3.2.2 First Session: Diagnosis and Psychoeducation

Introduction
The therapist starts the first session in the following way:
a) Introduces himself or herself (name, profession).
b) Explains his or her interests (the purpose of the present project/mission).
c) Explains the ethical stance.

The patient has a right to know who the therapist is and what his or her motivations are. This initial phase and the way the therapist presents himself or herself and his/her work, is already a crucial trust-building step between therapist and patient.

> **Example:**
>
> My name is ... I am a psychologist (nurse, social worker) from the organization ... (clinic, nongovernmental organization, university, school). I am here to assist people who have experienced extremely stressful conditions such as war (rape, forced migration, torture, massacre, accidents) and to document the human rights violations that have taken place. I usually work at vivo's outpatient clinic ... (in a treatment center, in a hospital) with survivors of violence / refugees / from various countries. We hope to use what we learn from you to improve the way survivors of violence are supported and respected in the future.

Always invite and encourage the patient to ask any additional questions he or she might have.

Pretreatment Diagnostics
Because this manual deals with the treatment of PTSD and related disorders rather than with how to diagnose PTSD, we will not go into the details of clinical interviewing. It is evident, however, that establishing a clear psychiatric history and correctly diagnosing PTSD with the use of a structured interview require extensive theoretical and practical training and skills.

To ensure whether an individual has PTSD or not, it is not sufficient to rely on a self-report instrument. A structured interview by an expert is mandatory. It is important to not just measure the occurrence of PTSD symptoms, but also the quality, frequency, and intensity of these symptoms. It is necessary for the therapist to have a good, reliable sense of the individual's condition and complaints. Since we know that many PTSD patients also suffer from comorbid disorders, commonly occurring conditions such as depression and

> **Useful diagnostic instruments for PTSD**
>
> Some currently used instruments that have been developed to measure psychiatric disorders and PTSD:
>
> **CIDI** – Composite International Diagnostic Interview (section M, interview & diagnosis according to DSM-IV and ICD-10; developed by WHO) (WHO, 1997).
>
> **CAPS** – Clinician Administered PTSD Scale (interview & diagnosis according to DSM-IV; also measures severity and intensity); currently the gold standard.
>
> **SCID** – Structured Clinical Interview for Mental Health (PTSD interview & diagnosis according to DSM-IV).
>
> **PDS** – Post-Traumatic Stress Diagnostic Scale (self-report measure filled out by the patient; measures the frequency and occurrence of PTSD symptoms; can also be applied in interview form [PSS]). (Foa, 1995).
>
> **UCLA PTSD Index for DSM IV** (self-report or interview; child, adolescent, and parent versions; measures frequency and occurrence of PTSD symptoms; diagnosis according to DSM-IV).

drug addiction should be screened for as well. While depression may recede with NET treatment, drugs are often self-prescribed as a means not to think about the events and, as such, hinder processing of the memory as required by NET. PTSD diagnosis always includes an event checklist that screens for typical traumatic event types. Such an instrument provides the therapist with an overview of the traumatic history of the patients, and what events might appear within the narratives. Event checklists for survivors of violence can be found in Appendices B and C.

When introducing the preliminary assessment to the patient, explain that you have brought a set of questions with you that will cover symptoms that many survivors often suffer from. Explain that it is necessary to gather this information to get a better idea of what the person is experiencing and that it will help you to establish a diagnosis. You should also be sure to mention that while some items may apply, others may not. Before you start the interview ensure that the person has understood the importance of answering each question. Finally, reassure the patient that all answers given will remain confidential.

If the presenting patient does not meet the criteria for PTSD, it is necessary to decide what treatment modalities, other than NET, are available to help the person with his or her trauma. NET, so far, has only been evaluated for patients who meet the criteria for PTSD.

Psychoeducation

After the initial interview and diagnostic assessment, the respondent will be interested in learning the results. If the person suffers from PTSD, it is advisable to continue with psychoeducation immediately following the diagnosis. Initial patient education includes explaining the patient's condition such that he or she understands the diagnosis. It is important to explain to the patient that trauma symptoms are a common response to extreme and harmful experiences and that violence causes not only injuries to the body, but also to the mind and the soul. Most people suffering from PTSD symptoms feel relieved when they hear that there is a well-defined concept for their condition, that they are not "losing their mind" (as they might fear themselves), and that these wounds to the soul can be healed, although scars may be left.

Continuing with the psychoeducational component, explain to the patient that the symptoms, although a common response under such horrifying experiences, are not serving a useful purpose and are only leading to continued suffering. Explain that memories of the trauma are intrusive occurrences, which may come in the form of visual images, single sensory perceptions, or other more complex internal states, into the mind and body. Explain that these intrusions keep the person in a state of vigilance as long as the trauma is unresolved. The unprocessed material thus requires conscious processing, which will occur within the therapy. Once the incidence is successfully filed or stored in memory as part of the complete personal biography of the patient, the symptoms will decrease.

Summary   Psychoeducation should include these elements
• **Normalization** (it is normal/understandable to have such reactions after a trauma);
• **Legitimization** (the symptoms experienced today are the result of responses from the traumatic situation);
• **Description of trauma reactions** (including related symptoms);
• **Explanation of the therapeutic procedure** (imaginative exposure & habituation, narration, and a step-by-step explanation of the therapeutic process).

1. Psychoeducational example of *normalization:*

Anyone would be distressed after what you have experienced. This aftershock is known as a posttraumatic reaction. The human brain is designed to promote sur-

vival. Therefore, our mind and body are made in such a way that they will perceive and store threatening information to a great degree. Because this happened to you, your body is in a state of looking for and predicting danger before it occurs again. It is far preferable for us vulnerable humans to be too cautious, too hypervigilant. However, this is a survival strategy which is painful and extremely exhausting, as you know. It is no longer needed now, as the threat you survived happened in the past.

2. Psychoeducational example of *legitimization:*

The problems you are experiencing now are not adaptive responses for your present life. In a life-threatening situation, people become highly aroused (no sleeping), danger-focused (not concentrating on other things), and numb (not feeling any pain in your body). During the event, your body and mind were in such an alarm mode (e.g., sweating, heart pounding, rapid respiration). This is a common state for your body to be in following a traumatic event. [use the particular symptoms of the survivor to explain]

3. Psychoeducational example of explaining the symptoms – *intrusions, hyperarousal, avoidance:*

No matter how hard survivors try to avoid them, memories will always come back. They enter into your everyday life, both at night and during the day. All of a sudden you may get upset, anxious, or detached from reality without knowing why. During a terribly horrifying moment, your mind cannot comprehend what is going on. It is just too much. You are overwhelmed by the bodily alarm reaction and anxiety. You are very aroused in order to react fast and ensure survival, but you have no time in these moments to process any of this information. However, your brain has a completion tendency: It brings up these feelings and fragments later in order to understand and digest and put together all of this, until it makes sense. Reliving those feelings, pictures, and bodily sensations indicates that the mind is actively attempting to process this horrible event, to make it understandable – because this may be vital throughout life. It causes these unresolved inconsistencies to reemerge into consciousness again and again. But you push them away each time, because they are so painful and horrifying. You avoid them. What you want to do is now to give them room here during therapy. We want to explore them together and eventually give your mind a chance to understand and integrate these memory fragments.

During the course of narration it is vital to show and verbalize your empathy and respect for the person and the tragic experience that has been lived through. Stress the wonder that the victim has managed to survive or that, e.g., she or he was able to save the children. Make this part brief but personal. Only mention positive things you truly believe in. Do not exaggerate. The patient might be struggling with survival guilt and belaboring this could exacerbate the negative feelings. If you make him or her a hero, he or she might not dare to tell you about the event for which he or she feels guilty or ashamed. The patient may end up hiding events from you. The therapist must not judge or evaluate the particular behaviors that led to survival.

It is advisable to work out your own way of explaining the theory behind NET to your patient according to the culture, age, education, experience, and worldviews of the individual patient. It is preferable to stick to the theoretical part of this manual. Children will need an unsophisticated but equally full explanation. It might be good to provide psychoeducation to children in the presence of their caretakers, so that questions can be addressed at the same time. Treatment, on the other hand, is often easier when relatives are not present.

Regardless of the type of patient education model being used, the main elements should result in the following:

- The patient should clearly understand what you are going to do and that he or she has voluntarily agreed to participate.
- The patient should understand what is expected of him or her in the process of NET.
- The patient should not be left with unanswered questions about the therapeutic activities and the techniques you are employing.

Most people do not have any experience with psychotherapy; some people may never even have heard of it. However, there is usually a concept of healer, elder, or counselor within every culture. It is very important to explain that this *healing journey* will only be possible when the patient is fully active in the process and fully aware of the procedure. The patient should understand that this is not a passive act performed by the therapist onto the patient. It is important to explain the possibility of an elevated fear level during the exposure process – these are moments the survivor has successfully avoided so far. Psychoeducation should answer questions such as: Why is the patient willing to seek treatment now? How can talking about the traumatic event help this person to overcome their suffering? Why is giving a testimony an important step in the healing process? These are questions the therapist may pose to the patient in moments of doubt or confusion.

4. Psychoeducational example of *explaining the interaction of avoidance, exposure, & testimony:*

This terrible experience left you with a wound that cannot heal properly. It has been hurting and bothering you ever since it happened. Just like an inflammation, every time you touch the past experience, it hurts. Therefore, as you have quickly learned, it is better not to be in touch with these memories of the past. However, when a surgeon cuts the wound and removes the infected tissue, it has the chance to heal. Some people would like the same thing done with their traumatic wound, and they ask us for anesthesia. Unfortunately, this is not possible. In order to alleviate the pain from this wound you must stay conscious and expose yourself to the memory of the traumatic events by reweaving those fragments back into your story and into your biography. When this is successfully completed, the symptoms will subside.

In order to successfully integrate the terrible things that have happened to you, we need to gain access to these past events. We want to look at all the thoughts, feelings, and bodily sensations you experienced during the incident. We want to explore them as completely as possible and go through the incident in slow motion. I know that you have tried hard ever since to erase these feelings. They have been terrorizing you and leading a life of their own within you. However, we do not want them to do this to you any more. At this time, we are going to face them together. Up until now, it may have felt as if you have been held captive by them. This is often exactly what the perpetrators wanted. They want that you will remain a prisoner of these horrible events forever. But we are not going to let this go on. We are going to do something about it. If you can manage to vividly remember those memories, feelings, and sensations you had during the incident of the event long enough, those terrible emotional reactions will eventually subside. They will lose their grip and the impact they are having on you. They will fade away.... I know it is hard to imagine, but I will help you and this can become true for you, as it has for many others. What has happened to you is a violation of your human rights. Our ethical standing is based on the Universal Declaration of Human Rights, where the international community has agreed on your right to have a dignified life. Nobody is allowed to violate or harm you. Through the process of giving testimony about what has happened to you, we would like to provide the chance for you to do justice through the documentation of what you saw and went through. Testimonies like this counteract forgetfulness, ignorance, and denial. (Your report will be furnished in a written form and, depending on your wishes and acceptance, can be used for documentary purposes and human rights work. However, the story of your suffering will be kept absolutely confidential if that is what you want.)

5. Psychoeducational example of *explaining the narration procedure:*

Through telling your story, we want you to construct a detailed, comprehensive, and meaningful narrative of the traumatic events in your life. The goal of having you retell the things that have happened to you is that you can reintegrate it into your and your people's life history. We want to fill in all the gaps and holes until your testimony is complete. We want you to retell it to us until some of the bad feelings about the events subside, until some of the pain dissolves, and until the fear has a chance to defuse. In our experience, the more complete the narrative, the more the symptoms will get better. We will always go according to your life's timeline. We will proceed in chronological order, step by step, as the events unfolded. After this, we will go over it again, correcting and completing things, as necessary, until we reach a final version within 10-12 sessions. However, each single session will always be taken to a point of completion. It will last about 90-120 minutes. We will take enough time at the end of each session to make sure you are comfortable with whatever came up during our work.

It is mandatory that you tell your patient clearly that it is common to experience fear and high levels of arousal when recalling the traumatic event during narration (Figure 10). Explain that the severity of the reaction to the traumatic incident is unknown until the memory has been retrieved. There may very well be surprises. It is part of the therapeutic work to uncover exactly how the trauma network is connected and which experiences are keystones in the brain's network. Reassure your patient that sessions are always taken to a point of completion and that whatever has been triggered in a session will be worked through to a point until the patient is comfortable again. Inform him/her that information processing may well continue even after the session has ended. There might even be a transition phase during which symptoms become worse. Reassure your patient that during the whole therapeutic procedure you will always be there. They must know

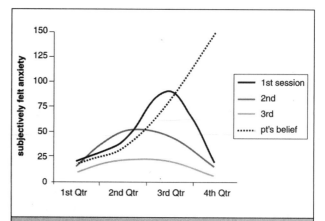

Figure 10. Change in subjectively felt anxiety across sessions: During the first session, the patient typically believes that fear and anxiety will increase ever more (represented by "pt's belief" in the figure). Explain that it will be like crossing a mountain, whereby a plateau will be reached, after which the fear will subside. The next time the mountain will be much lower, i.e., the anxiety level will climb less each time the narration is repeated and elements are added. A session must not be ended before the subjective and physiological arousal has subsided. Qtr = quarter period of each session.

you will always be there to turn to when difficult feelings arise in the session. In subsequent sessions, the therapist should always ask about what the patient experienced between sessions, and these topics should be addressed, as needed, in that session.

Do not forget to tell the person that nothing will be the same again once this therapeutic process has started. Our experience is that, as a result of the therapy, survivors will begin to feel different, think differently, take action or change their way of behaving – possibly even during the course of therapy. In addition, NET might have consequences on their social networks as well. As therapy survivors begin to dare to stand up for their rights, they often want to speak out. They rank and respect their own needs and conditions more sensitively, they refuse to tolerate abusive relationships, and some may even want to change their lifestyles. Yet regardless of whether any of this happens, exposure therapy is a personally very challenging intervention. While in treatment, patients need a warm, supportive, and understanding environment. During some sessions, the patient may require a particularly supportive social network. These times are usually during the second session (when the individual is first talking about the trauma), the third session (when the person is approaching and intensely working on the hot spot), and the forth session (when the person is beginning to process and integrate the difficult memories).

flowers - happy
resources

Stones - fear
- trauma experiences
- sad

3. The Therapeutic Approach of Narrative Exposure Therapy (NET)   43

3.2.3 Second Session: The Lifeline

After a diagnosis of PTSD has been established by a structured interview in the first session, and after psychoeducation has been provided, the lifeline is next, usually at the beginning of the second session. The lifeline has become a symbol for NET, because it represents the life "story" of a person in a ritualized and symbolic way. Hereby survivors lay out their path of life along a rope or string that symbolizes the contiguous flow of time. They place flowers for happy major events and good times in life – e.g., for positive, empowering occurrences, moments of achievement, for important relationships, experiences of bliss and acceptance, and so on. Flowers can serve as resources for life. Stones are placed as symbols for fearful and in particular for traumatic events such as life-threatening experiences, violent acts, abuse, combat experiences, rape, assault, injury or harm, captivity, natural disasters, accidents, etc. Survivors usually also place stones for sad or difficult moments in life, such as loss of a loved one or times of hardship (divorce, loss of a job), suffering, failure, as well as other stressful, unpleasant, and negative experiences that they have had to endure. The lifeline-process is started by a short explanation on the meaning of the "line" (a rope or string), the flowers (either you use real fresh flowers or plastic flowers in different colors, shapes and sizes – whatever is available in the particular setting you are working in) and the stones (you can use any stones from roadsides, mountain areas, riverbeds, etc., in different sizes, shapes, and textures). It is good to offer a variety of stones (large and small) and flowers, so as to give your patient choices for the representation of events. We suggest abstaining from introducing further symbols. Flowers and stones carry a clear message and give structure. We only allow flowers and stones as symbols for the lifeline to avoid watering down its clearness. However, 'fear'-stones have a different psychological dynamic and meaning than 'grief'-stones. In cases of loss, a small candle lit and placed on the stone may be allowed as an adequate symbol for the bereavement.

The survivor is encouraged to take the string or rope in his/her hand and lay it on the floor (sometimes on a table) according to the memorized "flow" of his/her own way of life. This is just a first approximation of how this line should be formed. Adjustments can be made as the process evolves. When the rope/string is put on the floor, the therapist encourages the patient to start placing the symbols on the lifeline. The patient starts with a first symbol for his/her birth, which is put down at the very beginning of the rope. The symbols are then placed in chronological order. The therapist

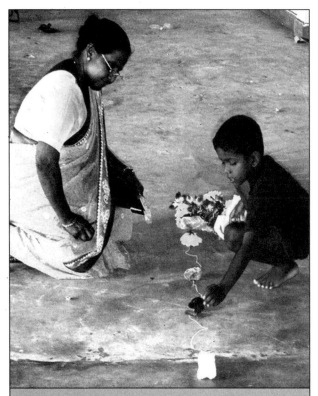

Figure 11. Laying the lifeline is essential for children and for adult survivors alike. (Picture taken by Dr. Claudia Catani, vivo international)

guides the patient to name and mark important events and turns in life (Figure 11). The therapist verbalizes and summarizes what he or she understands from the survivor's "life-map." It is important here to encourage the patient to give each symbol (flower or stone) a heading or name and to clearly pin it down in time and space. Usually a short sentence or a few words are enough to characterize an event or a lifetime period or a distinct event without going into detail (e.g., "16 years old, living in my hometown, I was raped by my uncle," "35 to now, living here in this town," "26 years old, birth of my first child, named Maria," etc.). Although we should not avoid naming clearly what each stone means, the lifeline exercise is not the time to actually confront the event. In some contexts it might be difficult to find exact dates of events. In this case, it is good to encourage the description of parallel events (e.g., "my first child was born in the year, when an earthquake was shaking our land"). Even if the year or age are not exact or not known by the patient, the main effort is placing symbols as much as possible in chronological order along the line.

Throughout the whole lifeline procedure, the therapist helps the patient to stay on the cold memory side *coldmemory - just facts*

(see Chapter 2.2) – i.e., the therapist helps to focus on facts, names, dates, etc., rather than on emotions, sensations, physiology, etc. This is important to ensure that during this work, the fear/trauma network is not activated, because full emotional engagement in the form of exposure to significant events will happen later in the course of therapy. The lifeline exercise is only an overview of important life events – a roadmap. In this regard, it is helpful to settle and cool down after each placement of a symbol, especially stones, before starting to talk about the next event. Otherwise, feelings pile up toward the end of the lifeline, and emotions get mixed up and confused. Helpful verbalizations to move the process forward are statements such as "Yes, I see this is a big stone. I understand that the death of your husband had a big impact on your life. We will take good time later to talk about this experience in detail. For today we have laid its representation on your lifeline. The experience has now got a place here. This was in 1998. You were then 58 years old and living in Rome, Italy. Let us move on from there and see how your life continued."

The line starts at birth and is laid out proportional to the age of the person (e.g., one half meter for every 10 years of age would make a length of 2 meters for a 40-year-old client). Make sure that a good remaining part of the rope stays coiled up, since this symbolizes the unfolded future, which is yet to come. Make sure you start and finish the therapeutic exercise of laying the lifeline in one session. It usually should not take longer then an hour, even if many events are there (Figure 12).

After the lifeline has been laid out, the survivor and the therapist take time to look at the *gestalt* as a whole and appreciate the important work achieved. Sometimes the survivors wants to contemplate the process of the laying, sometimes there are the first important insights on one's life as a whole or on interrelated events. The therapist wants to allow such emergence of meaning, but keep in mind that the whole story can only be evaluated once it is told. It would be far too early for interpretations and conclusions on the basis of this rough and often incomplete overview. Also, do not allow focusing in of the patient on certain events at this stage. You will not have enough time or possibilities for appropriate exposure in this session. Also, this process is hard work on the patient's and on the therapist's side, and after an hour or so, there are hardly enough emotional and mental resources left to zoom in on one particular symbol. It is important to end the session in a placable manner. This is not the time for complaints, bitterness, and grieving. In case these topics appear, the therapist can advise that first we want to have a detailed look at each single event in the course of therapy, and

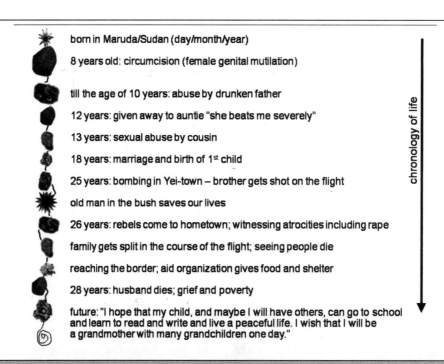

born in Maruda/Sudan (day/month/year)

8 years old: circumcision (female genital mutilation)

till the age of 10 years: abuse by drunken father

12 years: given away to auntie "she beats me severely"

13 years: sexual abuse by cousin

18 years: marriage and birth of 1st child

25 years: bombing in Yei-town – brother gets shot on the flight

old man in the bush saves our lives

26 years: rebels come to hometown; witnessing atrocities including rape

family gets split in the course of the flight; seeing people die

reaching the border; aid organization gives food and shelter

28 years: husband dies; grief and poverty

future: "I hope that my child, and maybe I will have others, can go to school and learn to read and write and live a peaceful life. I wish that I will be a grandmother with many grandchildren one day."

chronology of life

Figure 12. Lifeline of a Sudanese refugee woman. Flowers symbolize positive events, stones symbolize negative events (traumatic, stressful, or sad experiences).

work through them. Later, there will be time enough to evaluate the life and particular experiences as a whole.

At the end, children often like to make a drawing of their lifeline to include it in their narration document. For adults, we often offer to take a picture of the lifeline as long as it is laid out on the floor (or the table). The patient receives the picture as part of the written testimony at the end of treatment. Make sure as you go along to take notes of what is laid out in front of you and the meaning statements of symbols. Some therapists like to attach small Post-it stickers along the floor as the symbols of the lifeline evolve. Others just draw a simple replication on a notepad and add their own notes.

Finally the *therapist and the survivor together remove the lifeline* and place the objects back in the box. It is not advisable to leave the "life" on the floor of the therapy space when the patient leaves. Clients who have gone through the lifeline experience often report that they feel protective about their lifeline, and they do not want it to remain lying exposed in the room. The laying of the lifeline has to be accompanied with utmost respect by the therapist and other witnesses. Other than in survivors of multiple (different) traumatic events (such as robbery, traffic accident, war bombing, etc.), in some complex trauma patients, the lifeline is not very detailed or conclusive at the first attempt. Some survivors of childhood abuse, continuous trauma, or personality disorders are utterly unable to retrieve reliable memories of their past. This often results from severe dissociative responding when attempting to retrieve autobiographical memories. In fact this inability to recall is an indicator of severe traumatization. However, with all patients the lifeline exercise is carried out no later than the second NET session, as well as the patient can do it. There is no wrong or right. Within one session, the laying of the lifeline is completed, and in the following session the narration must begin. In cases in which the original lifeline deviates significantly from the final sequel of events as they emerge in the course of the narrative therapy, the lifeline can be laid out a second time at the very end of treatment as a closing ritual. In fact, in complex trauma patients (such as those who have suffered childhood sexual abuse, or who have suffered many, very similar rapes), this can be a much better final activity than reading the whole narrative again (as we would suggest doing in multiple trauma survivors who have been exposed to many different event types) (see Section 3.2.6).

In narrative exposure therapy with children (KIDNET), the child can lay the lifeline each time they come back

for therapy, as a starting exercise. This is possible because the life of a young child and therefore the life*line* is short, and the material can be placed in a short period of time. Naturally, with this brief review, the child gets a welcome opportunity to see where the session continues and to realize to what point the narration has reached and where to continue. For adults, with their much longer life and more complex experiences, this is obviously not advisable. But it is generally useful to have a photo of the lifeline or a sketch at hand at the beginning of each session so as to point out to the adult survivor during which lifetime period a narration continues, how much has already been accomplished, and how much yet remains to be worked on.

Summary Laying of the lifeline

Every NET starts with a life overview. Important biographical events and life changes of a survivor are symbolized in a ritual called "the lifeline." The lifeline, a standard element of NET, is mandatory in therapy with children, with illiterate clients, and with survivors of multiple or continuous trauma.

The lifeline exercise consists of placing positive and negative life events in the form of flowers and stones on a line (e.g., a rope) in chronological order. With the guidance of the therapist, the patient lays symbols while classifying them only briefly – just a label will do. The purpose of the lifeline is the reconstruction of subjectively significant life events in their chronological order. Since this is already a first look at the time and place when and where events happened within a life context, it serves as an introduction to the logic of the therapeutic process. The lifeline is a useful roadmap for the therapist; it helps in structuring the coming sessions and allows the therapist to foresee the "big" stones – namely, major traumatic events or very difficult life periods.

Warning: Avoid as much as possible the mix or confusion of memories from different events. Stay on the calm, cool-memory side with the patient while conducting the lifeline exercise. Do not mix in imaginative exposure elements into the lifeline session. Remember, the lifeline is not the narration itself. At this stage, it is NOT important to elaborate what precisely has happened. Identifying the events is enough.

Important rule: The lifeline exercise *must* be concluded within one session. It is not advisable to distribute the lifeline work over several sessions. Executing the lifeline as a form of incomplete and superficial exposure to traumatic material would be a severe mistake. This would result in the patient's fortified avoidance and heightened anxiety. Therefore, make sure there is enough time to complete the lifeline in one go.

3.2.4 Third Session: Starting the Narration

Preparation for the Narrative

The narration begins no later than during the third session (Figure 13). Once again, you should begin the session by briefly explaining what you are going to do together and by giving a clear timeframe to your work. You may ask your patient at this time if she or he has any remaining questions. Beware, however, that this may open the door to avoidance. Your patient might use question-asking as a way of avoiding rising fear and of delaying recall of the events. At the same time, patients are extremely tense, since they know that "it is going to happen today." They usually want to get the process over with as quickly as possible. For this reason, it is advisable to not waste too much time getting started. Help your patient get started by asking the question "so, when/where were you born?"

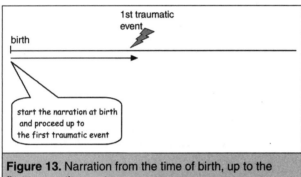

Figure 13. Narration from the time of birth, up to the first traumatic event.

Starting the Narration

The chronology of the narration should address all traumatic incidents throughout the course of the person's biography. This will likely proceed through the following stages: childhood – pretrauma (brief) – first traumatic incident (detailed) – posttrauma (brief) – lifetime in between (very condensed) – second and following traumatic incidents (detailed) – outlook for the future (brief).

Start the person's narration with their family background. Get a picture of how the patient grew up, what the relationship to their parents was like, and what other significant persons played a role in their life. Even during the pretrauma period, it is advisable not only to collect the facts, but also to encourage emotional processing. When the individual is narrating some event that was particularly pleasant or some minor stressful event, they can begin to practice processing the emotional content. Children particularly enjoy talking about happy times, but adults will also enjoy talking

about joyful moments of their childhood. For many people who have been exposed to organized violence and war, the memory of good moments in their life have disappeared together with the bad memories. This exercise in bringing up emotional content can be useful in training the patient to chronologically narrate an event. The patient can learn to include emotional as well as cognitive and physiological details. Try to get a feeling as to how these various experiences shaped the person's unique way of coping with stressful events, as this might help to understand the patient's reaction to the traumatic events. You might ask yourself the question: *Who* was this particular person when trauma struck?

The time you spend on the pretrauma period depends on the number of sessions that are available for treatment, the number of traumatic events in the patient's life, and on the life period in which the first traumatic event occurred. If this event took place in childhood, the amount of time you can spend talking about life before the event will be relatively short. However, do not spend much time on this period prior to the event. The patient has been psychologically preparing to talk about the trauma, and some survivors become impatient when too much time is spent talking about other things. On the other hand, some victims may attempt to extend the discussion of the pretrauma period so as to avoid discussing the difficult material. Just spend sufficient time on the pretrauma period to comprehend and validate this time period, but be aware of reserving enough time to discuss the first traumatic event during this first or second session. In the session in which you confront traumatic material, allow full expression of the fear response and afterwards give enough time for the patient to calm down when narrating the period that followed the traumatic event.

Narrative Exposure to a Traumatic Event

In this next portion of the manual, the NET procedure will be explained in detail. Each step is the same for every traumatic event the person has experienced. (See examples of complete narrations in Appendix D.)

Recognizing a Traumatic Event

One of the important steps about gathering the information from the narrative is developing the ability to recognize when the patient is discussing a traumatic event. There are different pieces of information that can be helpful in determining what is a traumatic event in the narration. As a first step, you can always rely on the information you gathered in your pretreatment diagnosis. The individual identified those events that were most traumatic in his or her lifetime. Use this diagnostic information as a tool, making sure to read over these forms before beginning the sessions. By being aware in advance of what the person experienced, you can be listening for clues that the patient is broaching difficult topics.

Another possible way of identifying when the patient is discussing a traumatic event is by how the person is speaking. Often, during NET, the way a person talks will change when they have been asked about a difficult time period or are coming to the point of discussing a traumatic event. These are some cues to look for:

a) *The person's report may begin to be more fragmented and incoherent.* When the thoughts are fragmented or incoherent, you might have difficulties understanding what the person is trying to tell you about that time period. Sometimes a traumatic event might even be completely skipped or left out of the narration. However, oftentimes the patient will drop a subtle hint about the trauma while attempting to avoid it or in having difficulty expressing it. For example, a patient might say: "Then, in 1998, the war came to our town. I lost my brother, we had to flee." If a patient gives this type of vague description with missing details, you should always ask for more information. In this case, you might ask the patient if he/she personally witnessed how his/her brother was dying or if there were moments at that time when his/her own life was in danger.

b) *You may observe that the patient gets nervous and emotional.* When the patient becomes too nervous or emotional, the narration may be interrupted. This may be due to intrusive memories that are coming to the individual's mind. The person may appear to be mentally absent or may be making general comments about his or her life rather than continuing with the narration. Be aware of the possibility of passive (dissociative) and active avoidance. If you notice this type of behavior, either absence or escaping, ask the patient if traumatic memories have come to mind. If the patient admits to experiencing difficult memories, and if these memories correspond to events from the time period in the narrative being told, then it is important to continue with the narration.

c) Once you have noticed that your client is approaching a traumatic event, then the major work of narrative exposure begins. Be aware that working with the client through the narration of a traumatic event will always take some time (at least 40-60 minutes) and that you should never interrupt this process. Only continue with this part of the narration when there is enough time left in this session to fully explore and discuss it and to allow for a full reduc-

tion of aversive arousal and fear by activating the autobiographic, the cold memories.

Assessing the Context of the Traumatic Event

When you get close to discussing a traumatic event, *clarify the period just before the incident* in order to enable the patient to embed it into the greater life story. The therapist must never work on the incident as a fragment of the person's life. It is key at this moment to orient the events and the speaker to time and place. Ask questions such as "where were you living at that time?" or "what time of the year/day/season was it when that happened?" and "were you already married at that time?" After getting a general sense of the time and place, then try and pinpoint the event even more precisely by determining the day.

> The following contextual information must be clearly narrated before you talk about the event in detail:
>
> **Time and setting:** Establish *when* the incident took place: Lifetime period, time of the year, time of the day, particular moment in the day (Figure 5).
>
> **Location and activity:** Establish *where* the incident took place. Where was the person at that time? *What* was she/he doing?
>
> **Beginning:** Establish the beginning of the incident. What point *marks the beginning* of this trauma or experience?

Starting to Narrate in Slow Motion

At this stage, the process of narration slows down. The therapist shifts to *slow motion* in time. Your patient's tendency will probably be to speed up even more and to jump to events further in the future. For this reason, it is going to take some persistence to keep the patient on a slower track. On the part of the patient, it is going to take some courage to slow down the recall of the event. At this point, even therapists experienced with traumatized survivors may begin to feel nervous and may want to avoid the difficult content and the increased signs of suffering of the patient. Learning to recognize this impulse will be helpful for the therapist, as it becomes an indicator that treatment is going well and that the patient is on the right track.

> At this point in time, make sure to:
> - Have survivor *imagine the beginning of the incident.* Begin to work through the incident from this point of the patient's imagination, viewing all of it in sequence.
> - Go in *slow motion!*
> - Help the patient to *focus on what was being perceived* during the traumatic incident (physical sensations, thoughts, actions at the time – ask for shape and color

of objects, types of smell, patterns of sounds, etc.). Support the processing of the material by following the emotional reactivity. Generate the physiology of that emotion: Pursue memorial association of the affect and generate memorial cues that elicit the physiological responsiveness.

- *Reinforce reality.* Prevent avoidance, dissociation, or flashbacks. Make sure that the person stays with you in her/his consciousness in the present time and talks *about* the past.
- Do not allow the patient to be taken back completely to the past in the form of a flashback. *Keep the patient grounded in the present.*

Place the incident within the context of the rest of that day. If, for instance, the traumatic event being described happened in the afternoon, start by asking questions about the morning on that particular day. Ask questions like: "Do you remember what you were doing that morning?" "Who was there?" "How did you feel?" "Was there anything special about this day?" and/or "What did you do next?" As you get closer to the traumatic moment, go more and more slowly, i.e., have more details reported.

As you get close to the time of the incident, ask questions that pertain specifically to the minutes and seconds prior to the incident. For instance: "So, you were sitting in front of the house with the fallen roof?" "You were walking on the right side of the gravel road at the time?" Help the patient to focus on those details that can be remembered. Again, sensory information is very important. Descriptions of sensory information include "I am aware of harvesting in the back part of the garden," "I was picking beans that I put in a wooden bucket," "I could smell the yellow flowers," "I saw the sun going down behind the village," or "I was busy thinking about my baby." Focus on the point that marked the beginning of the traumatic events. For example, the patient may say, "I smelled something burning" or "I heard a scream, and my sister was running towards the house" "It was suddenly very dark." Try to awake sensory memories. Ask your patient to place himself or herself at the beginning of the incident and to start going through the incident from that point, viewing all of it in sequence.

Example – The beginning of the traumatic experience

It happened at the end of the rainy season in that year. My son was 2 years old then. We lived on the south side of the village of N... close to the mountains. My husband was working in town at that time. I was in the house cooking that afternoon. I prepared rice. It was hot inside, and I felt a bit

tired. My cousin, who had been visiting me, had just left. We had been talking about water problems. All of a sudden I could hear shooting outside. (Narration continues....)

The next part of this incident happened outside of the village. The therapist again establishes the circumstances before the patient will be asked to place herself at the beginning of the sequence:

It was already dark, after sunset. I was running together with my son in the middle of the road. I am aware that my hands were too sweaty, that I could hardly hold my little boy. Even now when I tell you about it, my hands get wet. (Narration continues....)

Narrating the "Hot" Memory

The essence of NET is to connect the hot memory – i.e., sensations, feelings, and thoughts – to the corresponding sequences in the autobiography by putting all memory fragments into words and thus into declarative memory.

None of the processes by themselves are effective. It is not enough to let the patient just feel and reenact the traumatic experience without maintaining good chronological order within the narration. On the other hand, a good narration without an activation of all the elements of the fear/trauma structure (Figure 6), i.e., without emotional involvement, is also not helpful. It is important to be aware of both processes and to have the ability to switch between the two interventions and to support both elements. The NET process can be best understood as a spiral, which winds up toward the goal of a comprehensive, meaningful narrative of the traumatic incident.

The main procedure of emotional exposure within NET consists of two processes that must be present simultaneously:
(1) The hot memory (the fear/trauma structure) must be activated (Figure 14).
(2) The elements of the fear/trauma structure need to be put into words and inserted in the narration about the traumatic event.

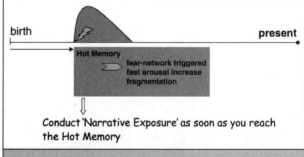

Figure 14. Upon reaching the traumatic event, the patient's "hot memory" is triggered.

> Be mindful of the following elements when encouraging the narrative process:
> Narrating – Reexperiencing in greater depth – Labeling in more detail – Integrating into the narrative again – Further narrating – Continuing this sequence

Interventions Used to Activate and Tag Hot Memories

The survivor might find many ways to avoid being exposed to the frightful experiences again. In these instances, the therapist must be both empathic and persistent, while being able to hear the worst of events without fear. Some patients may immediately begin to demonstrate noticeable symptoms of high arousal (sweating, trembling, heart beat), whereas other patients may be able to avoid any emotional involvement and stay surprisingly cool and calm. Others may show signs of dissociative responding. In all cases, the therapist is to ask questions about the contents of the fear/trauma structure. (However, see Chapter 3.3.2 for measures to take when the patient shows signs of dissociation).

Be aware that *hot memory* – the fear/trauma structure – consists of many levels: sensory, cognitive, emotional, and physiological elements (Figure 4). The activation of one single element or level can easily lead to the activation of other elements or levels. The therapist should be cognizant of addressing the fear structure on all levels. It is helpful if the therapist also imagines the traumatic situation in order to determine what might be salient elements. If, for example, a person saw grotesque scenes, such as mutilated bodies, it is most probable that the visual details of these scenes are a key sensory element of the fear structure. The therapist should ask for a detailed description of these images, even though the patient (and maybe the therapist as well) would like to avoid this. Keep in mind that if the images are in the fear/trauma structure, the patient sees these pictures in the form of intrusions anyway. It is crucial to try and help the patient put these images into words before they are given the opportunity to avoid them.

There are two types of interventions that help in activating elements of the fear/trauma structure:
1. *Direct questions:* With direct questions, the therapist can simply ask questions that address the elements of the fear/trauma structure across the different levels (Table 3). There are two ways to do this: Either in terms of the past or in terms of the present tense. The therapist might begin by asking the questions in the past, such as "What and how exactly did

Table 3. Example questions used to target elements of the fear/trauma structure across different levels of processing

Element of fear structure	Past	Present
Sensory	"What did the mutilated body look like?" "Could you smell the dead bodies?" "Could you hear the others screaming?" "Could you feel the gun in your back?" "Did you feel the pain in your legs?"	"Do you have the pictures of the mutilated bodies in your mind right now like it was then? What can you see?" "Can you see the soldier right now like he was then? What does he look like?" "Can you smell the dead bodies right now like you could smell them then?" "Do you feel the gun in your back right now like you felt it then?" "Can you feel the pain in your legs right now like it hurt then? How does it feel?"
Cognitive	"Did you think that you would die at this moment?"	"What did you think then; what now?"
Emotional	"Did you feel intense horror at that moment?"	"Can you feel the horror right now, like it felt then?"
Physiological	"Did your heart beat fast at that moment?" "Did you sweat a lot at that time?"	"Can you feel your heart beating fast right now, like it was beating then?" "Are your hands sweating right now, like they were sweating then?"

Table 4. Example of what sensory reexperiencing and labeling of emotional states may look like. In this case, the example of staying in touch with the perceptions is more important than the actual story.

Preceding this interaction is continuous narration up to the following crucial moment:

Patient: And then I was climbing that tree my brother sat on.
(Therapist can see that the patient's knees are trembling)
Therapist: How do your legs feel right now, when you imagine the climbing?
Patient: (astonished, looks toward legs) Well, the muscles are shaking a little in fact.... and my heart is beating fast.... I feel somehow weak.
Therapist: You are getting excited...?
Patient: Yes, I think it is because I know what is coming next. I had to climb higher up to get to my brother.
Therapist: Your body remembers the fear while climbing?
Patient: I have to do it.... But I am so afraid of falling ...
Therapist: In that moment you encouraged yourself to overcome your fear of falling. You said to yourself: "I have to do it!" meaning, you had to force yourself to go on?
(Therapist realizes that the hands of the patient form a grip that stiffens)
Can you feel the texture of the bark where your hands touched the wood?
Patient: Oh, my hands are sweaty, even now. I am afraid they won't make a firm hold! And this smell ... this is exactly the smell that reminds me of this situation again and again, each springtime....
Therapist: The smell of wet soil and fresh green?...And then you carried on climbing...?
Patient: (Silence)
I don't know.... I don't remember.... I am confused.
Therapist: Maybe your body knows? What do you feel?
Patient: I am shaking.... I should save my brother, but I can't.... Oh, no, it is like in a daze, I can't see any more....
Therapist: There was a fast heightening of arousal. You can even feel it now. It is hard to think clear in those moments. What did you see then, when you were in the tree?
Patient: I can see the leaves and the shade and the head and the arms of my brother hanging down from the tree. I see his face and I know that he can't hold on for much longer.... His face is stained.... His hands are clinging to the branch.... I don't dare move.

(Therapist realizes that the patient is in a 'fright' state of tonic immobility)
Therapist: How does your body feel right now, when you remember this immobility?
Patient: (takes time to get to the present feeling): I feel helpless and my body is paralyzed....
Therapist: Where?
Patient: (focusing on his perceptions): Only the arms, oh my arms ... I can feel them again ... Look, they are trembling and my legs too ...
Therapist: Exactly how they were trembling at the time on the tree. I understand, that you were panicky. You feared to fall to death.
Patient: It makes me so sad, that I coudn't help...(crying)
Therapist: You realized in that instant, that you were under life-threat yourself. It was impossible to move and help your brother. What a desperate situation!

Therapist comforts the patient as he cries. The patient now has overcome the immobility state. He is "defreezing" from paralysis and numbness. The emotions are perceivable and are labeled.
The person continues to narrate in great detail what happened next. How the brother fell from the tree. How the patient had to watch this, being helpless. How he heard the head of the brother hitting a stone on the ground. How he saw his brother lying there in the blood dying.... (etc.)
The patient tells the end of the scene. With the help of the therapist he talks about what this terrible experience and the death of the brother meant and means to him. Guilt feelings are confronted by the fact that the patient was in a tonic immobile state at the time on the high tree and that he couldn't move his body to help his brother. The therapist gives psychoeducation about the 'fright' stage during life-threat so that the patient can understand his physical helplessness (see Chapter 2.1.2. about the defense cascade and dissociation). In the next session the patient is invited to start to explore more details of the event, placing himself at the beginning and going through it again. He will integrate them into the existing narrative of what actually happened then, how he felt and now feels about it, and what he thinks about it today.

you feel when the gun was in your back?" However, when hot memories are activated, the individual often experiences the events as if they were happening in the present. In this case, the therapist may shift techniques and refocus the events of the present into the past. For example, if a patient experiences a strong sensation in the present, which is most likely related to a hot memory, then the therapist should relate it to the past. These sensations should never be left as part of the present. For example, if a patient reports that she/he feels a strong pain right now, ask her/him if it is exactly the same pain she/he felt during the traumatic event. This will help the patient to understand how the current experience was shaped by the traumatic event.

2. *Feedback of observation:* Some elements of hot memory – especially its expression in physiological and also behavioral responses – can be observed by the therapist. Direct feedback can be given about an observation such as "I can see your hands are trembling" or "your eyes are tearing up now." This will allow the patient to become more aware of these sensations and will lead to further activation of the elements of the fear/trauma structure. The therapist must not be afraid of feelings the patient verbalizes, of obvious physiological arousal, or of any behavior at any stage, as it reassures the patient that the therapist is accompanying him/her closely. There is no need for hesitation about attempting to label the patient's responses: experience shows that the patient will inform the therapist immediately, if the feelings have been labeled incorrectly.

The only task that the therapist has concerning the sensations felt and described by the patient is to help put them into words and connect them into an autobiographical flow, i.e., fit them into the narrative (Table 4). The therapist might invite the patient to perceive his or her own emotions without judging. This may be difficult for the person at first as they may still feel guilt or shame. The therapist shall be a model for this process by listening to the patient's experiences without judging.

It is important to trust the process of habituation. This continuous process of experiencing hot memory, while putting the elements into words and into a coherent narration will lead to habituation. Through this process, the emotional impact of the sensations and the physiological arousal will decrease. Initially, some emotions might be difficult to accept, such as rage, worthlessness, and guilt. However, the moment of exposure is the moment to experience the fear intensely. Therapist should not be sidetracked by the patient into a discussion about the adequacy or correctness of these emotions. This is not the time for cognitive interventions.

Interventions to Narrate
One way to monitor the therapist's own attentiveness to the storytelling is to try and imagine if a good movie could be made from the patient's descriptions. The patient's recall and explanations should be so detailed that it is possible to get a clear picture of what happened throughout the story. For the therapist, it is a good idea to try and keep this little film playing in one's mind. Most likely there will be gaps and inconsistencies in the narrative, which will become more noticeable when it is difficult to imagine what was taking place in the "film." At these times, it is the therapist's job to interrupt and intervene immediately. The therapist may want to say something like "maybe we can stop here for a moment. I am having trouble understanding what is going on in this sequence." Additionally, the therapist may try repeating as much of the story as he or she knows to the client followed by „and what happened then?" These interventions will help patients to construct a detailed narration and show them they are not alone in reexperiencing this process.

When the first hot spot is being discussed by the patient, the therapist might prefer to stop transcribing the narrative. It will likely take all the attention of the therapist's focus to handle the emotions and simultaneously keeping the narration going. As soon as there has been some habituation, the therapist may resume writing. The therapist might also recite aloud to the client what he has written down and understood at this time. Be sure to always use the survivor's own words and idiomatic expressions.

Interruptions Through Strong Sensations
Sometimes the narration is interrupted because the person experiences somatic reenactment and somatosensory intrusions, or intense bodily sensations, which she or he cannot understand or link to any event in that moment. Instead of talking about fear, it is important to stay with the sensory elements. You should assist the patient in getting in touch with the somatic experience, and give the patient the opportunity to find out what the feeling means or what the source of the feeling is. When the narration is caught in a hot memory, the therapeutic measure is to help the person become aware of what is happening and to help the patient sort through these perceptions. The therapist will help the patient trust her or his reactions and experiences, which might be confusing and seem to lack sense.

The first step is to identify the sensation. The therapist would assist with questions like:
- „What does this sensation feel like?"
- „Where in your body do you feel what?"
- „What quality does the sensation have (cold, warm, fast, slow, heavy)?"

From there, the therapist will help the person categorize these perceptions and integrate them into the narrative. To build up the patient's trust in his or her own inner feelings, the therapist will gently, but unwaveringly, proceed and reinforce the person, in whatever way he or she chooses, to get into contact with those sensations. The therapist will assure the person that whatever appears is perfectly all right and that there is no need to analyze or judge it. All of this can be done later on. Perceiving and describing the sensations are the priorities.

Example – How focusing on perceptions „tells" the trauma story

A man, who was witnessing a massacre, interrupts his narrative at one point. He had been bending forward in his chair for quite a while. Because he had been sitting like this for a while, he then noticed that his back was hurting. As he became aware of this sensation, he also noticed that he was experiencing a feeling of suffocation as well. In response to the therapist's question, "Where do you feel it?" the patient suddenly commented, "It is in the neck. And my heart is beating fast." The therapist encouraged the man to continue becoming aware of the perceptions and sensations of his body. Describing it more carefully, he mentions that it is very dark around him. The man begins to get very excited, and his body stiffens. He is hardly breathing. A few minutes later, still continuing to observe and name the sensations of his body, he realizes that the different elements of sensory information that he is experiencing come together to form a whole picture. It is a part of a traumatic scene he lived through. The man was in a panic during a traumatic incident, in which he anticipated getting killed if the persecutors found him. He was hiding for hours squeezed in a dark hole, completely focused on whether there were any footsteps coming closer. Now all of these bodily reactions made sense: a fast beating heart, being unable to breathe properly, a sensation of narrowness and darkness. The experience was then semantically integrated into the narrative, by putting words and meaning to the experience and to his bodily sensations. Other parts of his PTSD-related experiences, such as nightmares of being trapped in a cave, were also meaningfully connected to the scene.

Habituation

For a more in-depth discussion of this topic, please see the checklist for therapeutic detections to support emotional processing and habituation in Section 3.3. Challenging Moments of the Therapeutic Process – NET In-Depth, for when there is no habituation.

Habituation is the decrease in symptoms that occurs after being exposed to the stressor for a significant amount of time. The continuous process of activating and narrating hot memory will lead to habituation, which means that the emotional impact and physiological arousal decreases over time. A session should never be stopped before some habituation has taken place. In fact, there has been evidence that ending a session when the emotion is still at its peak level of intensity, only serves to aggravate the symptoms (Rothbaum, Foa, Rigge, Murdoch, & Walsh, 1992). Consequently, the length of time the patient is exposed to the recall of a hot memory must be long enough to allow the trauma to lose its emotional intensity. The arousal peak, or that highest level of emotional intensity around telling the event, must have been reached and a notable reduction in fear and excitement must have been present before a session should be ended. Figure 15 shows a successful and typical habituation process of an exposure procedure as felt subjectively by the patient and as can be measured with physiological indicators.

After habituation takes place, hot memory is transmuted into cool memory. However, full habituation

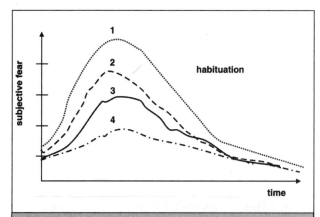

Figure 15. During the first emotional exposure, patients might have the perception that fear will increase infinitely. Initially, (1) fear will go up until it reaches a peak and decreases naturally. After a second (2), third (3), and fourth (4) emotional exposure, fear will decrease significantly, and habituation will settle in. When exposure is stopped while fear increases, e.g., by avoidance, before habituation can take place, a negative pattern of increased anxiety is likely.

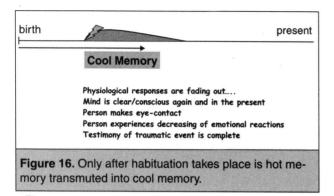

Figure 16. Only after habituation takes place is hot memory transmuted into cool memory.

cannot be expected after only one single session. Some fear reduction will take place within a single session as the patient is exposed to the traumatic life events in the telling of these events. As the habituation process takes place, the client's high level of arousal, originally experienced while addressing the hot memory, will come down from its highest point (Figure 16). Further habituation will take place in the following sessions, when the events are reviewed again. Habituation will continue to take place between sessions, as the patient will most likely continue to think about the event differently from the way they did before treatment. By the final NET session, the goal is to achieve the maximum level of habituation possible.

Note: The biggest mistake at the point of an elevating fear response during exposure would be to halt, interrupt, or avoid discussing the memory before habituation (or a feeling of relief) has occurred. During "exposure," arousal and negative emotions are going up. During "closure," arousal is decreasing, and the therapist supports calming down. Always be unambiguous in which direction you are going: **no mixture of exposure and closure!**

The Period Just After the Event Narration – Ending a Session

After the arousal has been reduced noticeably, be sure to bring the narrative to a close for this session. Even if time in the session is running out, it is of utmost importance to establish a clear ending to the traumatic event that has been worked on. The rule is: Never end a session with your patient in the middle of recovering a traumatic scene! The way to bring this closure is by moving on to the event that occurred immediately after it. To do this, the therapist tries to have the patient verbalize in at least a few sentences what happened in the time period following the incident. It is important to clarify the time period, whether it is in minutes, hours, or days, following the traumatic event, in order to enable the patient to integrate the incident into the

greater life story. The therapist might use questions such as the following: "When did it end?" "Where were you?" "What were you doing?" "What did you feel?" "Who was with you?" "What were they doing?" "What were your expectations at the time?"

The therapist thus begins with story-telling prior to the trauma, and proceeds to events occurring during the trauma and shortly after the trauma. This allows for the trauma to be placed within a context of time and space, and allows for the patient to grasp and sense the context surrounding the event. Before actually ending a session, the therapist will make an assessment to determine whether the patient's arousal level has subsided and to be certain that the person is calm again with a peaceful, positive, and relaxed feeling.

We can make sure of this by looking for the following signs (adapted from Bisbey & Bisbey, 1998):
- *The patient's emotional state is improved:* Return of normal face color, the patient is demonstrating and making statements that he or she feels better (relieved, peaceful, smiling); muscle tension and trembling has resided; the body position indicates a more relaxed internal state; and negative physical sensations have disappeared (pain, headache).
- *The patient's attention shifts from his or her mental environment to an awareness of external environment:* The person is making eye contact with the therapist, is noticing things in the environment, is aware of the passage of time, is aware of external noises, is feeling hungry. The patient may be commenting on activities that he or she will be involved in after the session, or patients may be commenting on things they have noticed about the therapist.
- *There is evidence of a cognitive shift in the patient:* The patient's thinking about the meaning of the traumatic experience seems to have changed. The patient states that she or he has achieved insight into the experience; the patient is making connections between the trauma and other experiences in her/his life; the patient is reporting that her/his experience makes more sense now. The patient talks about the meaning of the event. Finally the patient reports that it feels as if the trauma is over and is no longer as significant as it was.

This work should bring you to the end of your session. The length of a session depends on the person being treated. There are no fixed time frames for the length of sessions. Although the therapist may want to cover as much ground as possible, it is important to be sensitive to what an individual can process in any given time. Usually a session finds its natural ending within about 1 1/2 hours. Finish a session when it makes contextual sense (for example, after you have worked through a chapter of the biography) and depending on the therapeutic process and the patient's progress in the session. This is better than setting an artificial time. The best moment to "fade out" a therapeutic session is when there is enough emotional distance from the last exciting and arousing hot memory. Never start working on a new hot spot when there is not enough time to complete the process of exposure and habituation.

Cognitive Restructuring and the Days After

At the end of a session, after some habituation has taken place, patients often use this cooling-off period to make sense of the trauma and to put meaning to the trauma. More formally, one would want to support this *cognitive restructuring* process (Figure 17). The following issues often arise after exposure to the memory of the events:

- The patient might have some *new insights about the meaning of the event* for her/his life. Often patients realize how the everyday emotions and unhealthy behavioral patterns (such as general anxiety, mistrust, rage, outbursts of anger) have their origins in the traumatic event.
- The detailed narration often leads to a *more thorough understanding of a person's behavior during the event*. This might help to modify resulting feelings of guilt and shame, as the person might realize that he or she had no other choice at that time.

The next logical step would seem to be comparing the once hot memory to the now cool memory and discussing the implications of this transition with the patient. However, this step can be postponed by the patient until the beginning of the next session. Many survivors need time to realize the impact of an exposure session. A good part of the cognitive processing and emotional evaluating happens after the exposure session – without the presence of a therapist. Much of the beneficial process of increased awareness of what has happened

takes place between sessions. When the therapist and patient meet again, the therapist should be open to positively receiving any thoughts and considerations the patient might have had since they last met. The therapist may want to explain to the patient again that this process of coming to new realizations is a natural sign of processing information and is a first step toward healthy development. If a patient wants to talk about these issues, the therapist can support the process by reinforcing a change to more adaptive beliefs.

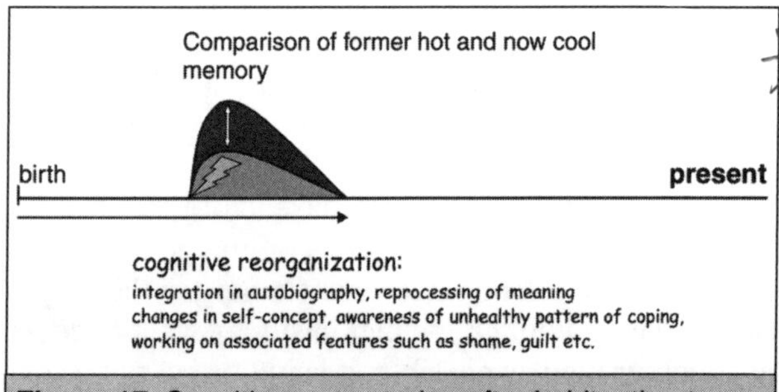

If the survivor brings it up, ethical issues or human rights topics can be addressed with the survivor. Subjects such as regaining one's dignity or potential actions that might be taken, such as political involvement, may very well arise. The patient may also bring up other topics related to healing, such as joining a self-help group or seeing some alternative therapist (someone who performs body work, massage, or other alternative practices).

Scheduling a New Session

Following the first exposure sessions, a series of processing steps will occur in the patient. Thoughts or feelings that the person had previously been avoiding may surface. The individual facing these thoughts or feelings may experience more unrest than usual or may suffer from an increased sensitivity to cues triggering the fear/trauma network. Patients may find themselves feeling more angry or irritable than normal. It is important to inform the survivor about the possibility that these experiences might take place, and it is equally important to inform the person that this is a completely normal response, one that is an integral part of the healing process. Your patient may want to start keeping a diary and or jotting down anything that they observes. The life of the person will start changing – not just internally, but also in interactions with others or in day-to-day behaviors.

Because of the intense nature of the work being conducted and the processing that is necessary, sessions should not be scheduled too far apart from each other. One to two sessions a week seems ideal. Less than that is possible, but some patients might find greater lapses in time difficult to cope with. With clients who have reported severe traumatic incidences at different periods in life, it is particularly important to agree on when the next session will be. This will prevent the avoidance that leads to prolonged suffering. The only exception in terms of a short time between sessions is with the last session. It might be useful to schedule the last session 2 to 3 days after the next to last session. This intentional break will give the patient time

Comparison of former hot and now cool memory

birth   **present**

cognitive reorganization:
integration in autobiography, reprocessing of meaning
changes in self-concept, awareness of unhealthy pattern of coping,
working on associated features such as shame, guilt etc.

Figure 17. Cognitive restructuring after habituation to a traumatic event.

to evaluate and rethink the entire testimony process. In between sessions, a lot of cognitive and emotional processes will take place for the patient. Ask your patient to watch out for those processes and possible changes, so that you can start the next session by talking about them. As stated earlier, exposure processes not only occur during, but also between, therapeutic sessions, and alter the associations within the fear/trauma structure.

Tenses of the Narrative – The Emotional Impact

While working on the incident during the therapeutic session, the survivor should process the material in an optimal state of arousal. We want the client to get emotionally involved in the controlled reliving of the event. Usually a breakthrough is achieved, when the person is finally able to feel intensely and when he or she becomes really emotional about the scene. However, reliving always must be "as if" only: We want the person to process the past emotionally, while being grounded in the present. The person should never be hurled back into the factual scene without keeping a strong bond to reality.

- When underengaged: use the present tense to make the scene more vivid and to get the full activation of the fear/trauma network (e.g., "You are lying on the floor right now.... Can you feel the hand on your body now? Where do you feel it touching?...").
- When overengaged (or panicky): use the past tense to achieve a lower level of autonomous activation, to reinforce reality, and to point out that it is over (e.g., "Take a moment and experience [feel] how you are sitting on this chair now in the room with me here, while we are thinking about that moment in the past, when he had his hand on your ...").
- Explicitly compare *then* and *now* responses, sensations, emotions, and cognitions during the session (e.g., "Your heart was beating in that moment then, how is it now?...").

The written testimony is always furnished in the past tense, while sensations and feelings that are produced by the story are put in the present tense.

Levels of Parallel Processing During NET

There are different processes going on in parallel that need the therapist's continuous monitoring during and between NET sessions:

1. The incident: what happened then, at the time of the incident (past)?
2. Here and now: what happens now during the session?
3. Present: what is going on currently in the life of the patient, and how does it influence the therapy?

4. The narration and the narrative: during the session and when updating the testimony.
5. The therapeutical contact: how are "we" doing during and between sessions?
6. The therapist: how am "I" doing during and between sessions?
7. Cognitive and emotional reorganization: during and between sessions
8. Admin: timing, appointments, etc., during and between sessions

Following all sessions, the therapist's homework is to write a first draft of the patient's life narration up to the point at which the narration stopped.

3.2.5 The Following Sessions

When meeting at the beginning of each session, it is important to be observant of the emotional condition the patient is presenting with that day. This will reinforce the certainty in the patient that you are a reliable and attentive companion in this difficult period of life recall. A therapist must not say things like "You are depressed," since this is to label a person negatively without actual knowing whether it is true. Be aware that in a helper's position, a therapist has quite some power over a patient's beliefs. It is always better to speak about one's impression, without judging, to use "I messages," and to verbalize carefully. One way of starting might be to say, "I can see that your hands are trembling." "How have you been since we met last?" or "I notice today that you look tired and exhausted." "Have you had trouble sleeping these past nights?" Or you might address something you notice in the patient: "I can see that you are restless." "Is something making you nervous/bothering you?" or "Could it be that...?" A few minutes at the beginning of the session can be taken to explore and label the emotional state in which the patient finds herself/himself. Of course, once the patient is settled, the narration proceeds (Figure 18). At this point, your focus is on the lifeline. Beware that it might be tempting to avoid it and prefer to talk about other topics that are pertinent, yet off-task, such as how the patient is coping or how the patient is handling daily problems. Avoidance and with it a conspiracy of silence between client and therapist has many subtle faces.

In the second session and every session thereafter, the written narrative from the previous sessions will be re-read – sometimes in abbreviated form – to the patient. Where appropriate, the patient will be asked to fully imagine and relive again the incidents with the purpose of correcting and detailing the report. The purpose of this is that the testimony and the habituation process become more and more complete. Reading parts of the document (make sure the person is aware of the relevant lifetime period), once again facilitates emotional processing and exposure in the same way as described above, until arousal decreases when memories of a particular event are recalled. Ask about changes in your patient's perception. "Did you feel different this time when we talked about the traumatic incident?" "How about your heartbeat? How was that?" "What were you feeling this time?" In this way your patient starts to build up personal awareness about emotional and cognitive changes within herself/himself. When you come to the end of the document, continue exploring the person's life further. Simply proceed along the autobiography. Do not be tempted to return or go backwards in time, but always move forward (remember that you can bring up past issues in the beginning of the next session). During this process, it is possible that a second traumatic event will emerge (Figure 18). By going through this step-by-step process of reading back the narrative to the patient and having the details filled in, an entire narration or eyewitness testimony will be completed, including all traumatic events of that person's life in chronological order (Figure 19).

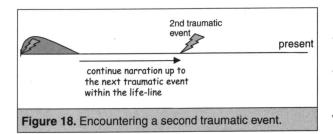

Figure 18. Encountering a second traumatic event.

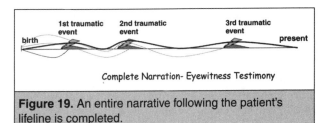

Figure 19. An entire narrative following the patient's lifeline is completed.

3.2.6 The Last Session

In the last session, the report is read to the patient, and all final corrections are made. Again, the therapist must make sure that the criteria for closure are reached. In the final NET session recalling the testimony/narrative should have lost its arousing impact. The patient

might look at the narrative with a sense of distance (it's a sad but true story) or might look at this document as a tool for peace-building or educational purposes. Occasionally, patients take their narratives lightly when they are reread to them, making some comment such as "It is kind of strange listening to my own words. I realize that my perception has changed a lot...It's hard to imagine that I ever felt like this...." Some may see it as an important personal growth experience.

Finally, the patient, the translator, and the therapist sign the written testimony. The signed document is handed to the patient. If the patient agrees, another copy is kept for scientific documentation purposes. Upon the patient's request, a testimony, in anonymous form, is passed on to a human rights organization for documentation work. Sometimes survivors of childhood abuse want to refer the narration to a lawyer for possible judicial issues.

In contrast to surviving multiple traumatic events during one's life (e.g., first a circumcision (FGM), later during childhood a car accident, then several physical attacks when adolescent, then years later an earthquake, and bombing during a war when in mid-life etc.), in complex trauma, the patient has been exposed to the same type of traumatic stressors (e.g., sexual abuse) over and over again. When the full narration that covers many of these very similar events is read to a survivor, there maybe the risk that the events will fuse again, instead of further supporting segregation of the memory traces of the different traumatic experiences. In these cases, it maybe helpful to construct the lifeline a second time, as a closing ritual instead of rereading the whole narration which might activate the hot memory again. In these cases, after the last traumatic event is worked through in NET manner, the final session consists of laying out the lifeline (stones and flowers), now again in chronological order, at the end of treatment and naming the biographic events/symbols, that could be remembered and revisited during therapy. Often there are much more symbols on the lifeline compared to the first one at the beginning of therapy. In many of these survivors, the first lifeline that has been elaborated at the start of the NET will be lacking most of the events. Survivors of complex trauma with a high tendency of shut-down reactions, e.g., fright, flag, and faint dissociative responding, cannot explicitly remember many of the worst events they had to endure until before their fear-networks could be activated and they engage in exposure treatment (for dissociative shut-down see the defense cascade, see Figure 1; Section 2.1.2) at the beginning of treatment. When deciding for a final lifeline session at the end

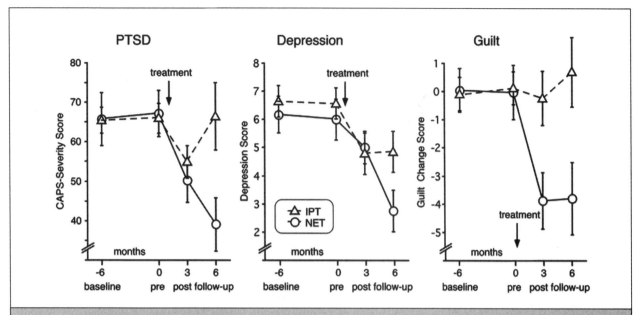

Figure 20. Time course (baseline to follow-up) for Clinician Administered PTSD Scale (CAPS) severity score, depression score, and change in guilt prior to treatment and in response to NET or group Interpersonal Treatment (IPT) (from Schaal et al., 2009). Note that the NET treatment but not the active control group showed a lasting reduction of symptoms (posttraumatic stress disorder [PTSD], depression, and guilt).

of treatment, the closing ritual here – much more as in a rereading-session, where the 'testimony' aspect is pointed out – focusses on appreciating and 'seeing' the biography of the survivor as a whole, the great work that has been completed now working through all of these memories, the importance of including all of these stones in the lifeline, which had not been possible in the first approach but now is, and which took a lot of courage. It is a quite ritualistic and dignifying moment, when looking at the Gestalt of the life of the survivor together at the end of treatment (see Section 3.2.3).

3.2.7 Posttreatment Diagnostic Sessions

Posttreatment diagnosis includes the evaluation of symptoms using the same instruments as prior to the treatment. Ideal times for evaluation are 6 months, and 1 year posttreatment. Diagnosis makes little sense earlier than 4 weeks posttreatment, as symptoms must be taken into account over a period of several weeks. What you would anticipate seeing over time, of course, is symptom remission to a degree where PTSD is no longer diagnosable. NET initiates a healing process that requires months, if not a year to fully unfold. Figure 20 presents a typical time course of symptom remission in response to NET, which indicates the change across the first half year posttreatment. It also shows the stability of symptoms across a 6-month pretreatment baseline. Data are from Schaal et al. (2009),

a randomized controlled trial in Rwandan survivors of the genocide that included a group Interpersonal Treatment for comparison. Figure 21 shows the effect sizes for the treatment of refugees and torture survivors at our outpatient clinic (controlled comparison NET versus waiting list control).

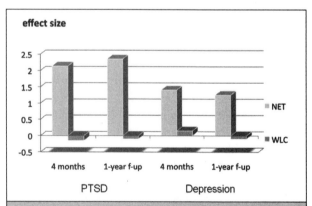

Figure 21. In a randomized controlled trial, survivors of organized violence who sought help at the vivo outpatient clinic were randomly assigned to a waiting list control (WLC) or a narrative exposure therapy (NET) group. The latter was applied during eight sessions, and two sessions were added for future-oriented counseling. As illustrated, effect sizes for posttraumatic stress disorder (PTSD) symptom remission and reduction of depressive symptoms are very large (f-up = follow-up).

Results from seven treatment trials in adults, have demonstrated the superiority of NET in reducing PTSD symptoms, compared with other therapeutic approaches. These studies also demonstrated that further improvements had been made at follow-up, suggesting sustained change had occurred. Emerging evidence suggests that NET is an effective treatment for PTSD symptoms in individuals who have been traumatized by conflict and violence, even in settings that remain volatile and insecure. NET is unique in that it effectively reduces PTSD symptoms in the individual while bearing witness to the atrocities endured (for review see Robjant & Fazel, 2010).

Today we know about *plasticity*, – how the brain's function changes its structure, and, vice versa, the structure determines its function (Schauer et al., 2006; Schauer, Elbert, & Neuner, 2007). *Challenge psychotherapy* receives innovative input from neurobiology (Aldenhoff, 2009). Basically these structural and functional changes in the brain should be measurable as a change with treatment.

Significant healing processes extend way beyond the PTSD symptoms proper. After successful treatment, trauma patients for instance might be able to go shopping in a crowded mall, may begin wearing skirts and earrings after decades of hiding physical appeal behind bulky clothes, will be able to meet friends, have a coffee at a public place after years of isolation, may be able to establish a relationship, can apply lotion on their body without feelings of disgust, may experience moments of sudden joy, or take a walk in nature, etc. Too often these very significant changes in life, the real-world outcome, so to speak, has been neglected by the systematic trials.

Summary   Most important rules of the NET procedure

- Never stop a narrative exposure session (emotional processing during exposure) during the height of fear and anxiety.
- Stay with the patient in the trauma narration until arousal has subsided.
- Prevent de-realization, dissociation, and avoidance.
- Prevent the patient from going back and forth in time while narrating.
- Do not mix *exposure* and *closure*. The therapist must know which of these separate actions is intended at every moment of the session.

Exposure = Fully reliving the events of the trauma scene. Staying in the traumatic incident until arousal and negative emotions subside; habituation and integration are achieved.

Closure = Ending the exposure situation and closing the remembrance of the traumatic scene. Supporting the client and helping them calm down until the arousal level has returned to normal.

3.2.8 KIDNET: Narrative Exposure Therapy with Children

PTSD Treatment for Children

In recent years, a number of investigations from various war zones all over the world have reported significant rates of PTSD in children exposed to acts of organized violence and war (see Kinzie, Sack, Angell, & Clarke, 1989, in children from Cambodia; Saigh, 1991, in Lebanese children; Somasundaram, 1993, Elbert et al., 2009; Catani et al., 2010, in Tamil children from Sri Lanka; Dyregrov, Gupta, Gjestad, & Mukanoheli, 2000 and Schaal & Elbert, 2006, in Rwandan adolescents; Thabet & Vostanis, 1999, 2000, in Palestinian children from Gaza; Papageorgiou et al., 2000, in children from Bosnia-Herzegovina; Karunakara et al., 2004; Ertl, Pfeiffer, Schauer, Elbert, Neuner, 2011; Ertl et al., 2010, in Sudanese refugee and Ugandan host children; and Catani et al., 2009, in children from Kabul, Afghanistan). Investigations conducted by the organization vivo in Sri Lanka exemplify the consequences of traumatic experiences and resulting PTSD in children. In an epidemiological survey, in which a representative sample of 420 Tamil school children in the then Liberation Tigers of Tamil Eelam (LTTE)–controlled Vanni Region of Sri Lanka's northeast were interviewed, we found that 92% of the surveyed children had experienced one or more severely traumatizing events, such as being caught in a combat situation, being in a situation of bombing and/or shelling, witnessing the violent death of a loved one, among others. Of those, about a third of the children (29% of the total sample) suffered from severe and chronic PTSD (Elbert et al., 2009), often comorbid with depression and somatization. Just as in adults (Schauer et al., 2003; Neuner et al., 2004a), we saw a significant relationship between the number of traumatic events reported and the number of difficulties children reported in social and emotional functioning. Factors such as frequent headaches, sleep disturbance, altered memory function, loss of ability to concentrate and pay attention, decline in school performance, loss of trust, and social withdrawal strongly impacted those children diagnosed with PTSD, limiting their chances for future healthy development.

Sri Lanka was also among the countries badly hit by a terrible tsunami in December 2004. A month after the disaster, we assessed symptoms of PTSD in 264 children who lived in severely affected coastal communities in regions that had been differently affected by the civil war: Manadkadu – northern coast (war zone), Kosgoda – western coast, and Galle – southern coast of Sri Lanka. As expected, the likelihood of PTSD symptoms was not only explained by the severity of the tsunami exposure and related family loss, but essentially depended on previous exposure to traumatic events. The results demonstrate that the individual trauma history determines the risk for developing PTSD in response to a disaster, such as the tsunami (Neuner, Schauer, Catani, Ruf, & Elbert, 2006).

In terms of trauma, the same is true for family violence, maltreatment, and abuse. It is known that heightened stress in childhood accelerates many forms of mental and physical illness. As suggested by studies in humans and clearly demonstrated in animal models, the impact of severe stress during development may leave an indelible imprint on the structure and function of the organism and the brain in particular (McEwen, 2002; Teicher et al., 2002). Besides PTSD, the psychological consequences of traumatic events can lead individuals into social isolation, hostility, depression, and substance abuse, and can foster somatization (Teicher et al., 2002). A significant relationship between childhood trauma and personality disorders, as well as other psychiatric disorders later in life has been postulated (see Section 2.1.3).

Narratives in Children

Humans form many fundamentally important emotional networks in (early) childhood. These memories will have lasting impacts on the individual behavior. They may, however, be only implicitly stored, and thus not be verbally accessible. In general, the capacity for autobiographical memory develops with age. Although infants and young children process and retain information (Bauer, 1996), events occurring before the age of 2-3 years cannot be recalled in narrative form. Due to developmental limitations, young children are thought to have problems with explicit memory functions and lack the competence for higher order memories (Williams & Banyard, 1999).

There is no doubt, however, that even very young children will remember traumatic experiences in an implicit way. In very small children, memories for traumatic events may be encoded differently, partly at a somatic and sensory, partly at an emotional, level ("the body keeps the score"), as opposed to the verbally mediated level (Bremner, Krystal, Southwick, & Charney, 1995). Due to the presence of threat, traumatic events are usually implicitly remembered, even in early

childhood, and the memories can be remarkably accurate (Koss, Tromp, & Tharan, 1995). In very young children (age 2-5 years), who cannot perfectly express themselves in coherent narratives, but who remember fragments, the memory nevertheless was shown to be accurate and correct (Howe, Courage, & Peterson, 1994; Jones & Krugman, 1986; Peterson, 1996; Terr, 1988), even when the traumatic event had taken place a long time ago (Widom & Shepard, 1996; Widom & Morris, 1997; Wagenaar & Groeneweg, 1990). Misperception and forgetting significant aspects of the experienced violence and horror are also common.

An active attempt to help children embed the traumatic experiences into their life context is useful in that it helps the child understand and integrate these traumatic experiences (Tessler & Nelson, 1994). In narrative exposure procedures, children are asked to describe what happened to them in great detail, paying attention to what they experienced in terms of what they saw, heard, felt, smelled, the movement they recall, and so on – as well as what they were thinking and feeling at the time. Initially the session is distressing, but if it is long enough to allow habituation, distress will fall, and more and more details will be recalled – just as in adult therapy. It was shown that after only four sessions of exposure, scores on intrusion and avoidance symptoms dropped dramatically (Ruf et al., 2010; vivo international, 2003; Yule, 2001). Additional pharmacological drug treatment has not been shown to be beneficial; in fact, drugs might even be harmful to the developing brain.

Even though children from the age of 8 years on are perfectly able to work with narrative exposure techniques, parents and teachers initially report that children would not easily talk about the trauma. Recent experience has shown that many children easily give very graphic accounts of their experiences and are also able to report how distressing it is to live with the related symptoms (Misch, Phillips, Evans, & Berelowitz, 1993; Ruf et al., 2010; Sullivan, Saylor, & Foster, 1991; vivo international, 2003). Although child survivors, like adults, feel an urge to talk about their experiences, paradoxically they usually find it very difficult to talk, especially with their parents and peers. Often they do not want to upset their caretakers, and so parents may not be aware of the extent of their children's suffering. Peers may hold back from asking what happened in case they upset the child further; the survivor feels this as a rejection. Often, however, children's traumatic narratives rely on co-constructions with parents or other adult caretakers helping to complement the story. Co-construction can assist the child in clarifying details of the traumatic experience, understanding its context and meaning, and addressing cognitive confusions (van der Kolk, 1996). Of special note, co-construction can address "pathogenic beliefs" that emerge out of inaccuracies and misattributions. It should be mentioned that parents and teachers are important models and interactive partners throughout the posttraumatic adaptation. However, in forced migrant populations it is likely that the parents have undergone the same traumatic experiences as their children. Therefore, they might bring their own avoidance to the therapeutic process of the child.

In summary, parents' and caretakers' involvement and participation in therapy has been shown to be a predictor for treatment success (Deblinger, Steer, & Lippmann, 1999; Steil, 2000). It is important to involve children at the right stage of the process and with adequate preparation. In any case, the informed consent that caretakers give to allow child therapy is a good entry point for psychoeducation. It is also necessary and important to respect the child's wishes concerning the parents' degree of involvement in their own narrative process.

Summary   Children and PTSD

Children are highly vulnerable to stressors that accompany war and conflict. Many studies have shown that children emerge from violence – familial or organized – with a number of mental health illnesses and serious psychosocial problems, including PTSD and depression, whereby both cause reduced daily functioning (see also Section 2.1.3). The child's right to a healthy intellectual, emotional, and social development is thus denied.

KIDNET – Utilizing the Lifeline With Children

The organization vivo has been developing a child-friendly version of NET, called KIDNET. Clinical trials have been carried out in Uganda with refugee children (Schauer et al, 2004; Onyut et al., 2005) and in Sri Lanka with formerly displaced children in the northeast of the country, and under the direction of Martina Ruf and Maggie Schauer at the vivo outpatient clinic of the University of Konstanz in Germany (Ruf et al., 2010). A full KIDNET testimony can be found in Appendix D.

In our research with children from different cultural backgrounds, ages, and levels of cognitive ability, we have generally been surprised at the extent to which children have been able to explore their life events, feelings, and thoughts associated with trauma. The key element in therapy with children is to gain and deserve

the trust of the young patient. Because it is not as easy to gain trust with children simply by talking, as we do with adults, we often use theater, illustrative materials such as figurines and drawings, in addition to the lifeline exercise, during therapy. Play and creative media can help children express their experiences. For example, we may encourage children to act out their traumatic experiences in role-play by requesting such actions as "show me how you sat on the ground when the car came" or by helping them recall details through painting. The therapist might ask, "Can you draw the expression on the man's face?" "Can you draw a picture for me that shows the house that you lived in and what it looked like?" or "Maybe you could show me in your picture exactly where the soldier was and where you were." Some of these elements, especially the replay of the body positions when the traumatic threat struck, are sometimes useful in psychotherapy with adults as well.

Since the lifeline exercise is a key feature of KIDNET treatment sessions, it will be described in more detail below. This exercise is especially important for the first NET sessions with a child. It helps to break the ice quickly and employs creative media, which allows the child's life story to unfold in a playful manner. In fact, this simple technique works so well that we have also been able to use it successfully with adults from many different cultures, especially when it is difficult for the person to reconstruct a clear chronological order of his or her life events.

Lifeline with children

Present the rope to the child. Explain that it symbolizes her/his life, with the beginning of the rope marking her/his birth. Ask the child to lay it out on the floor, leaving a good part of the rope unfolded to represent the future. Mark the point of birth and the present. Do not be surprised if the child lays out the lifeline across the space given or between obstacles. That's okay. Just ensure that it is clearly visible and accessible. Now show the flowers and stones to the child. (Ideally present a mixture of stones and flowers varying in size, color, and shape, to represent larger and smaller life events.) Explain to the child that the flowers represent happy moments in life, and the stones stand for difficult, fearful, or painful ones. Ask the child to place the flowers and stones along the lifeline. This will take a bit of time. Watch the movements and placements of the child closely. There might also be some backward and forward shifting of objects going on – make a mental note. When the child is finished, start at the time of birth and get an explanation for each flower and each stone placed. Make sure that a chronological order is established. Sometimes this means shifting objects around with the child until a proper timeline is established. After all major events, both happy and sad, are represented on the lifeline, ask the child to make a drawing of this lifeline. When they are finished ask them to give a name or a sentence to each flower and stone they have drawn, and write down what they say, including a brief note on what event this flower or stone represents. This drawing will serve as an important tool for knowing where the key moments are located in time and space in the child's life. Once you get into the narration, more events, both good and bad (more stones and flowers), might be revealed. That's fine; just ask the child to include them in the lifeline drawing. At the end of therapy, you can ask the child to draw the final version of the lifeline and to extend the lifeline further. Encourage the child to include some plans or hopes for the future. A final drawing can be encouraged in which the child draws future plans and hopes, such as "When I get married," "When I live in a house," "When I become a nurse or a doctor."

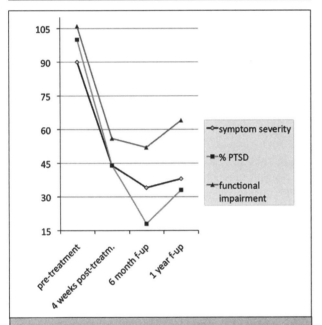

Figure 22. In a randomized controlled trial, children were randomly assigned to a treatment as usual or a KIDNET group. The latter was applied during eight sessions. The time course of outcome variables is shown only for the KIDNET group, as the control group received the active treatment after a 6-month waiting period. A pronounced reduction of symptoms and improvement of functioning continues throughout the first half year posttreatment in response to KIDNET treatment. Thereafter, children who continue to live in asylum seeker homes with continuing threat of violence and actual familial violence may show a worsening of symptoms. The symptom severity was determined by means of the UCLA PTSD Index with frequency rating. For illustration purposes, the ordinate shows scores ×2. PTSD diagnosis followed DSM-IV criteria (data from Ruf et al., 2010).

Three treatment trials and one pilot trial of KIDNET have shown KIDNET to be effective in reducing severe PTSD among children (see example in Figure 22). One further trial suggested the therapy may also usefully treat childhood traumatic grief. In a randomized clinical trial with severely traumatized refugee children at our clinic, Ruf et al. (in press) demonstrated significant treatment success on all PTSD-relevant variables for the KIDNET group, but not for the controls. The KIDNET treatment not only showed a clinically significant reduction in symptoms and but also a considerable improvement in functioning. This success remained stable at 12-month follow-up. The outcome for the control group demonstrated that, if left untreated, PTSD in children may persist for an extended period. With KIDNET, it is possible to effectively treat chronic PTSD and restore functioning in traumatized refugee children in only eight 90-minute treatment sessions. This success corresponds to the one obtained by Onyut et al. (2005) in an open trial conducted in an Ugandan refugee camp.

3.3 Challenging Moments in the Therapeutic Process: NET In-Depth

There are some typical problems that we face when conducting exposure therapy with survivors of violence. Others have already tried to highlight some of these critical issues (Bisbey & Bisbey, 1998). The following description may serve as an opportunity for a deeper understanding into how to accomplish the NET procedure.

3.3.1 The Patient Attempting to Avoid

Even after careful and sound psychoeducation, it is very likely that a patient may want to avoid this difficult and painful process. As explained earlier, the memory of trauma causes extensive distress to the victim, and so the patient might try to avoid confronting the traumatic material. Avoidance strategies vary from person to person. Some will speed up their narration and lose awareness, others will directly refuse to talk about a subject, others will try to sidetrack the discussion by changing the subject instead of sticking to the traumatic event. The goal of all of these strategies is to interrupt or avoid the exposure process. Reliving the trauma through imagination, however, is thought to promote habituation. Once habituation begins to occur, the individual will learn that anxiety does not need to remain forever and that avoidance or escape is not necessary to alleviate the anxiety. The therapist, although already having explained this during the psychoeducation phase, may need to explain these mechanisms again if avoidance is occurring (Figure 15). There are two steps to dealing with avoidance: First, you should openly acknowledge the patient's attempt to avoid, and validate that the process is painful and that you understand the desire to avoid. Second, you should explain that you are required, as the therapist, to notice and point out when the patient is avoiding. You may then explain that as a team, the two of you will work together in close cooperation to prevent avoidance. In some treatments, it may be necessary to intervene in this manner several times.

One reason for avoidance may be that your patient is unsure you will be able to handle hearing her/his story. Most survivors have never had an opportunity to share their story, or have never dared to talk fully about their experiences. This holds true for adults as well as children. It might be important to tell the patient about your own experiences. Tell your patient that you have worked as a researcher, therapist, social worker, nurse, or teacher in the field of counseling, human rights violations, or organized violence, as it applies to you. Share with them the fact that you have worked with refugees, torture victims, survivors, or that you yourself have experienced and overcome war situations or violence, if this is the case. Assure the patient that you know how to assist others in overcoming their suffering. Make sure that you continually demonstrate to the person that you can deal with whatever comes up. This is what you are here for: To accompany the person, side by side, back to the most horrifying moments of her/his past life. People who are afraid of hearing or imagining the atrocities that will invariably arise may fail as therapists in this setting.

3.3.2 The Patient Spaces Out: Dissociation

As explained earlier, some victims may have learned how to disengage from their traumatic emotions, sensations, and cognition. They might have developed unhealthy strategies in order not to feel the pain and threat (see Neuner et al., 2002, for a case vignette). The therapeutic challenge with NET is to look at the traumatic past from the present perspective. Reliving does not mean allowing the patient to be taken back to the past, as with a flashback. On the contrary, therapeutic exposure must enable the patient to face past events and to withstand the emotional distress these memories cause to a conscious mind in the present re-

ality. Anything else is not assisting the healing process. Allowing dissociation to happen will only strengthen the avoidance mechanism and increase anxiety. It is of major importance that the therapist helps the patient stay in the present.

The posttraumatic fear/trauma network may be activated through narrative techniques – e.g., when survivors report parts of their experiences. This will also activate the related support physiology of behavioral responses that have been engaged during the traumatic experience (Lang, 1979, 1984; Lang, Davis, & Ohman, 2000). Hence, we postulate that any activation of the trauma-related fear network will facilitate action replay of the defense behaviors the survivor has undergone peritraumatically. Patients who experience sympathetic activation in response to the stressor will not dissociate, whereas those who go down the whole defense cascade (Figure 1; Section 2.1.2), ending in parasympathetic dominance during the trauma, will produce a corresponding replay of physiological responding when reminded by a cue. The actual individual cascade of defense stages a survivor has gone through during the traumatic event will repeat itself every time the fear/trauma network – which has evolved peritraumatically – is activated again, i.e., potentially also during exposure therapy (Schauer & Elbert, 2010).

When survivors of severe violence first speak about the trauma, we can literally see that their hearts race, their hands become sweaty, and their breathing heavy. Those who experienced multiple and extreme trauma, however, may soon stop responding physiologically and report that they feel numb and unreal. Therefore, any trauma-focus approach, including NET, which is necessary to overcome the trauma-related disorders, requires the management of dissociative stages (fright, flag, and faint – Section 2.1.2).

We believe that self-injury is a means to induce relief through the initiation of vasovagal shutdown (Schauer & Elbert, 2010). By self-injurious behavior, patients may achieve tension reduction and mood elevation from stress-induced aversive states or anxiety (Bohus et al., 2000; Klonsky, Oltmanns, & Turkheimer, 2003). Based on their model presented in Figure 1 (Section 2.1.2), Schauer & Elbert (2010) have suggested that self-mutilating behavior facilitates tension relief through setting in motion the flag state. Self-mutilating behavior serves to initiate dissociation in the form of flaccid immobility. When mutilating the skin surface (i.e., cutting), a vasovagal reaction is launched. During this "shutdown," blood pressure and heart rate will drop, together with a fading emotional tension and a termination of ruminating thoughts, worries and troubles, etc. The potentially reinforcing effects of self-injurious behavior may account for the failure of some treatment regimens.

When the survivor responded peritraumatically with vasovagal shutdown or even fainted during the event, a replay of these responses and emotions during treatment, will quickly result in therapeutic failure. The patient cannot properly hear and see the therapist any longer, is not capable of narrating and reacting, is disabled with regard to responding and moving, and incompetent to reprocess emotion or cognition (Schauer & Elbert, 2010). During treatment, patients with the dissociative shutdown form of PTSD need assistance to actively fight the replay risk of vasovagal dominance (i.e., loss of blood pressure, bradycardia, vasodilatation, and eventually fainting). Instead, activation (active motoric engagement) may help to maintain arousal and prevent immobility. Relaxation techniques at that point are contraindicated since they would aggravate the cardiovascular problem and support fainting. During the first few times when confronting such a fear/trauma network, recall of the trauma material should be paralleled with forced reality testing, and therapists should actively engage in directive guidance, the very moment signs of flagging or fainting appear (for specific interventions, please see box below).

Characteristics of events that may elicit dissociative fright, flag, or faint are, according to Schauer & Elbert (2010) (for experimental confirmation of this model see Schalinski, Elbert, & Schauer, 2011, and Gola et al., in press):
a. imminence of threat/aggressor and total helplessness, e.g., direct body contact with the perpetrator, fixation (constraint), skin contact, danger of skin penetration (specially sharp objects – e.g., teeth and knife);
b. rapid arousal peak, often with startle, due to unexpected and sudden proximity of threat or aggressor;
c. presence of fresh blood, mutilated bodies;
d. being contaminated, having contact with infectious material such as mucosa and body fluids, including sperm, urine, or feces;
e. anal, vaginal, or oral penetration of the victim;
f. severe pain being inflicted on the victim;
g. and total helplessness, e.g., women or children with fewer means to fight back, or fixation of victim.

From this list of events, one can easily see that the experience of sexual abuse, where strong disgust reactions are often involved, clearly fulfills criteria for eliciting dissociative shut-down reactions. While threat heightens information processing and physiological arousal, it has been shown that, contrary to stimuli that elicit arousal and fear, disgust information is processed in the brain in a suppressed sensory perceptual and attentional way. This is akin to the central ecological function of disgust to minimize contact with contagious objects to avoid contamination and disease. At the physiological level, disgust tends to activate parasympathetic responses, reducing heart rate, blood pressure, and respiration, thereby suppressing action (see Krusemark & Li, 2011). Conversely, fear swings these systems in the opposite direction by stimulating sympathetic pathways, prompting fight or flight (see the inverted u-shape function of the 'defense cascade' in Figure 1, with its two presumed subtypes 'uproar-PTSD' (sympathetic-action PTSD) and 'shutdown-PTSD' (vagal-dissociative PTSD; Schauer & Elbert, 2010). Despite being both threat related, fear and disgust engage opposite mechanisms with contrasting behavioral consequences.

How do we notice the onset of dissociative shutdown during exposure? When confronted with traumatic material, there is – at least initially – a brief increase in sympathetic arousal, the uproar branch is activated even in survivors with shutdown PTSD types. During a period of agitation, heartbeat (palpitation) and blood pressure are rising, vasoconstriction (cold hands, pale face), and elevated emotional and physiological arousal can be observed. However, bodily numbing along with slight paralysis mainly in the legs are signs that dissociative shutdown stages are to be entered soon. Sudden yawning in the middle of the arousing exposure may indicate that hypotension has already set in (note: this does not mean the yawning at the end of exposure, indicating that actual relaxation has kicked in). The hands become warm due to vasodilatation, and the skin may change slowly from pale to red. The patient reports dizziness, blurred vision, and weakness of the muscles. The three main areas of behavioral changes that characterize a shutdown reaction peritraumatically can also be observed later, when recalling the traumatic experiences (Schauer & Elbert, 2010):
1. Functional sensory deafferentation: Incoming stimuli seem not to reach beyond the gates in the thalamus, stimuli are perceived as weak, distant, and unreal. During treatment, the patient may become unresponsive, with unfocused gaze;
2. Reversible palsy (stiffening because of heightened muscle tonus) leading to visible decrease of bodily movements and immobility, posturing, and finally waxy flexibility also during treatment;
3. Inhibition or disconnection of areas responsible for language processing and production of speech (unclear/confused speech, fragmentation of sentences,

inability to speak, almost no or belated response to acoustic stimuli).

Measures to counteract dissociative shutdown during the exposure therapy session: Before starting exposure with a shutdown-prone, i.e., dissociative patient, it is important that the blood sugar level is within the normal range. Shutdown reactions such as fainting and bradycardia may also be aggravated by low fluid volume from a lack of water, low sodium intake, and dehydration. Therefore, make sure that the patient is in an overall sufficient nutritional condition (be aware of eating disorders in complex trauma patients!) and has had an adequate meal that day; drinks may be offered in the clinic.

Following explicit psychoeducation on the causes of shutdown reactions during recall, the therapeutic measures which are likely to be applied during the exposure session must also be explained and consented to by the patient. At the first signs of a shutdown process, active mobilization and explicitly induced sensory contrasting of the time and place contexts (past versus present) should be initiated by the therapist in parallel with the encouragement of recall of the traumatic event. Feared stimuli can be presented briefly, always interrupted by reality testing, so that a vasovagal syncope will not be elicited. For survivors with shutdown PTSD, we suggest continuous shifting of attention between trauma-related material and the present context by recalling reality, sensory stimulation in the here and now, and motor activation using applied muscle tension and physical counterpressure maneuvers. The therapist should respond to prodromal fainting symptoms by engaging in context-contrasting and muscle tension techniques to counteract the incipient syncope. Active muscle tension appears as the treatment of choice for inducing significant blood pressure increase. Slowing the rhythm of the attentional shifts between the present and the past will allow the patient to process the trauma narrative unhindered by prior flag or faint responses.

In case of fainting or collapsing, the therapist should prevent patients from hurting themselves, by protecting the head during the fall. The patient should be placed on the ground with the feet elevated. A second person should be called to assist. The therapist should also lower herself or himself to the ground. The therapist will then start to establish a sense of reality for the patient, as described above. The therapist must be prepared for a change in behavior when the patient regains consciousness. The person may be disoriented or confused, or may be very anxious and emotional. Be prepared for any of the above.

3.3.3 Social Emotions: Shame, Social Pain, and Guilt

Usually, fear is the most intense emotion when working through the hot spot of the traumatic event, as it leaves strong traces in the hot memory. However, many victims of traumatic events report other aversive emotions in addition to fear, such disgust, shame, and helplessness. Although the major focus of most NET treatments is the fear of the most threatening part of the traumatic event, the NET procedure not only focuses on fear but on all emotions that were and are associated with the traumatic event.

The aversive, trauma-related emotions that occur in the patients' everyday life as well as during treatment can be divided into primary and secondary emotions. Primary emotions consist of sensations, cognitions, and physiological responses that had been present during the traumatic event and have been encoded as associative emotional reactions in the hot memory just like fear in the fear/trauma network. For example, disgust is a common reaction during gruesome scenes involving blood and mutilation. Disgust can be connected to the associative trauma network. Correspondingly, reminders of the traumatic event – e.g., seeing raw meat – may later provoke strong disgust responses.

In contrast, secondary emotions were not present during the traumatic event and are not directly encoded as elements in the fear/trauma structure. Rather, these emotions occur as a response of appraising the trauma story from the retrospective view that emerges during treatment. For example, during the narration, patients may become aware of the things they have missed during their traumatic past and hence become sad. Guilt feelings about actions the survivor has taken or has opted not to take in the course of the traumatic experiences are a common secondary emotion that was not present during the event but developed days or even years later. Sometimes, secondary emotions play a role in avoidance. For example, concentrating on ruminations about loss or guilt in everyday life or in treatment may help to avoid the intense emotions of fear or helplessness, which are usually much harder to tolerate.

The differentiation between primary and secondary emotions is not always easy and may only be determined as the NET procedure progresses. In a well-guided narration of the traumatic experiences, all primary emotions that were present during the exposure to the traumatic stressor should be felt and noticed. All aversive sensations and cognitions have to be un-

Practical examples for countering dissociation (from Schauer & Elbert, 2010):

	Therapeutic intervention when uproar is dominant during the exposure session *Activation of elements of the fear/trauma network in relation to their autobiographical context (space and time when event has happened)*	Therapeutic intervention when shutdown is dominant during the exposure session *Activation of elements of the fear/trauma network in relation to their autobiographical context, supported and interrupted by continuous reality testing and cardiovascular activation* *sensory stimulation* *encouragement of speech production* *until trauma material can be processed without shutdown.*
Sensory-afferent	Emphasize the exploration of sensory details of the *past* traumatic event, comparing or contrasting with sensations and emotions in the present during recall.	Emphasize the exploration of sensory details of the past traumatic event, comparing or contrasting with sensations and emotions in the present during recall + stimulation of the senses in the *here and now*, e.g.,: present positive fragrances (e.g., lemon), offer tasting probes (peppermint oil or chilli-gum), switch on bright light, present tactile information (e.g., texture, ice-packs), direct attention to auditory stimuli in the here and now.
Motor-efferent		Emphasize activation of the skeletal muscles, enhance blood pressure and muscle tonus (above all, use applied tension, physical exercises, leg crossing, physical counterpressure maneuvers), and use body balancing tasks.
Language processing	Emphasize the narration of the *past* traumatic scene	Emphasize the narration of the past traumatic scene, supported by the facilitation of continuous narrative engagement in the *here and now* (e.g., active communication; enhanced speech production).
Emotional processing	Support the full emotional expression	Support full emotional expression allowing and promoting specifically anger affect that has been inhibited peritraumatically.
Nutritional demands		Pay attention to adequate nutrition (caution for malnutrition/eating disorders); increase dietary salt and fluid intake in daily life; advise to drink 500 mL of water (approx. 500 mL if tolerated) just before exposure to trauma material.

Counteract and abstain from:

• Termination of exposure before contextualization and integration can take place (i.e., avoidance)	• Termination of exposure before contextualization and integration can take place • Disengagement from the here and now • Relaxation (instead of activation) • Sensory similarities between the trauma context and the therapeutic setting • Stimuli that are associated with disgust or similar to body fluids and feces (i.e., ammoniac) • Threat cues in the here and now (instead: present safety signals) • Semidarkness in the room and objects for hiding (e.g., large plants, sitting behind furniture)

derstood from the perspective of the person in the narration and embedded in the autobiography representing the past context of the person. However, certain primary emotions, for instance, shame, are related to interpersonal processes and require special attention of the therapist to prevent a disruption of the treatment process.

Difficult Interactions – Social Emotions

Whereas fear indicates a threat to the body and life of a person, other primary emotions relate to threats that occurred in interpersonal interactions. For example, shame can result from degradation and humiliation from parents or peers (Mills, 2005; Tangney, Stuewig, & Mashek, 2007). Such emotions indicate that not primarily the physical, but the social integrity of the individual has been threatened. The ongoing lack of responsiveness of a caretaker or direct verbal abuse by others can threaten the attachment to the care provider, the group membership, or the social rank of an individual (Mills, 2005). Social violations of this kind are common among survivors of child maltreatment who report a history of emotional abuse (Egeland, 2009). But also many forms of organized violence, most of all torture, aim at harming the social integrity by making the victim feel dependent, inferior, and ashamed.

For animals living in social groups, a threat of social exclusion may be as dangerous for survival as a direct hazard to bodily integrity. As a consequence, evolution has equipped humans, like other animals, with an automatic defensive system that reacts to social threats (Panksepp, 2003). Presumably, this social defense system was built upon the phylogenetic older fear cascade and somatic pain system. Social threats trigger the same fight–flight reactions as physical threats in terms of hormonal and physiological responding (Macdonald & Leary, 2005; Williams, 2007). Following social threats, flight reactions occur in the forms of social withdrawal, hiding, and submissive gestures, whereas interactional fight reactions consist of superiority signals, anger expressions, overt aggression, and threats of payback and revenge.

Consequently, social emotions, together with their physiological and cognitive components, can become strongly tied to prototypical cues that indicate a potential threat to social integrity. For example, repeated verbal abuse and degradation by parents can produce a shame network which associates cues of abuse with behavioral impulses of hiding. Features of these situations may include sensory elements of all modalities. Cues range from a pejorative or aggressive expres-

sion and face, to a hostile tone, abusive words, or to messages that are felt as rejection. Repetitive experiences of a variety of these cues will lead to a generalization of stimulus features until eventually a wide range of interpersonal situations will automatically evoke stress responses of the defense cascade. Consequently, many situations will bias attention and interpretation such that the threshold for feeling threatened becomes very low, i.e., the respective trauma-related associative networks may be activated by interpersonal situations that might be very different from what had been experienced during the exposure to the traumatic stressors.

The power of these associative structures to determine behavioral responding depends on their size and the strength of interconnections among its items. These are determined by the frequency of aversive social experiences during the life of a person, and by their behavioral relevance, usually coded as intensity of affective responding to these experiences. A long history of social rejection, neglect, and humiliation involving different close persons can lead to the establishment of a widely generalized structure that might have a lasting impact on almost all social encounters later on. On the other side, the availability of a single responsive and accessible caretaker or a close connection to a peer group may be protective and prevent the formation of strong memories of aversive social situations. Rejection experiences are less threatening for individuals who are attached to a protective and responsive caretaker or who can rely on other forms of social support.

In the long run, large and strong sensory-perceptual representations of social aversive situations can lead to a variety of psychopathological phenomena. Many survivors of emotional abuse and rejection report vivid intrusive recollections of prototypical situations. However, the devastating nature of social trauma occurs in relationships with other people. Strong associative networks result in different forms of dysfunctional interactive behavior, including impulsive aggressive reactions, avoidance of social interactions, and mistrust. As emotional abuse and rejection typically occur repetitively, at a daily rate even, the formation of a temporal and spatial context for each single experience is usually not possible. As a consequence, there is the danger that networks of social aversive emotions will remain unconnected to autobiographical context. Then the victim will show pathological behavior even toward people not related to the trauma and in situations that may be much different from the original abusive context.

Shame

Whenever we know, or suppose,
that others are depreciating our personal appearance,
our attention is strongly drawn towards ourselves,
more especially to our faces.
Charles Darwin (1872/1998)
The Expression of the Emotions in Man and Animals

Shame is a moral emotion that indicates that a person feels that she or he has transgressed the values of her culture (Tangney et al., 2007). In contrast to guilt feelings, which refer to single incorrect acts or decisions of a person, shame involves the conviction that the self of a person is not adequate to comply with the moral demands and social acceptability. As a consequence, the person has constant fear that her or his shortcomings could be detected, which would result in the ultimate rejection or loss of social rank. Furthermore, shame has a lot to do with the disapproving glance of the vis-à-vis: Being 'looked at' and not found a valuable, acceptable person, not having an adequate or even repugnant appearance in the 'eye of the other', is a major fear in all humans. In many cultures, the connotation of 'shame' is associated with nakedness and indecent exposure of body parts. Social phobics do not want to and avoid to be looked at, avoid eye contact and fear to arouse dislike and disgust in the other person, so that s/he turns away. The evolutionary roots of shame lie in the covering of private parts (genitals) and hiding personal hygiene (toilet training). There is a biological preparedness for shame in response to sexual activities and sanitary activities, which is already present in children. This is why traumatic events that include abuse, rape, sexual molestation, or the bodily fluids of another person, evoke intense feelings of shame.

Shame is characterized by a distinct expression, which includes a confusion of the mind, attempts to hide oneself, and submissive signals such as blushing, downward-cast eyes, slack posture, and lowered head with silence, and speechlessness. Moreover, shame-prone people are convinced that a disclosure of intimate details, exposing the inner self, bears the risk of being turned down. This behavior obviously poses a serious obstacle to NET. At the same time, shame can be accompanied by strong aggressive impulses or behavior that compensates for the threat of inferiority.

It is important to be aware that the spectrum of norms and values differs considerably between cultures and even within subcultures. The understanding of a person's shame feelings requires the comprehension of the norms of the respective community. For example, shame may result from not being able to meet standards of values such as achievement or duty. Perceived transgressions against the standards of self-control and attractiveness may cause strong shame. Often, victims of sexual violence feel that they have contributed to the violation of moral commands related to divinity and purity. Since shame has got to do with the 'eye of the other' it is of major importance that the 'look' of the therapist communicates validation for the patient at all times. Furthermore, cognitive intervention should include and confront the fact that the perpetrator is the one who should feel ashamed for what he did and loose social status because of his acts, not the victim.

High levels of shame-proneness are predicted by experiences of emotional abuse in childhood (Stuewig & McCloskey, 2005). Continuous hurtful words and humiliations on the background of a lack of parental responsiveness interfere with the confidence to comply with the norms of the society. Shame causes the victim to attribute the responsibility for a perceived transgression to herself or himself rather than to the offender. Extended periods of dependency between victim and offender bring about a strong tendency to attribute the violations to oneself, as any attempts of blaming the perpetrator would increase the risk of further punishment or neglect. In these cases, the development of self-blame, self-criticism, and even self-hate may be a safe but painful way of coping with the maltreating environment (Gilbert & Procter, 2006).

Social pain

Social pain is an intense aversive emotion that results from violations of the social integrity of a person, including exclusion, rejections, separations, grief, and bullying. Social pain is a condition that is at the core of a variety of related emotions including sadness, heartbreak, loneliness, and yearning (Macdonald & Leary, 2005). All of these conditions either indicate that the relationship with a person or a group has been damaged or signal that the desired relationship to a person could not be achieved. The intensity of the pain depends on the strength of the discrepancy between the desired and the actual closeness. Recent research has shown that social pain is an intense emotion that is characterized by similar sensations and physiological processes to physical pain and that it is accompanied by a strong stress response. Like other strong stress responses, experiences of social rejection can trigger intense fight or flight reactions, including social withdrawal, but also excessive or impulsive aggression. Just like shame, repeated experiences of social rejection is a predictor of aggressive behavior in children, adolescents, and adults.

The repeated experience of exclusion and rejection can lead to the inclusion of social pain in sensory-perceptual representations. It is likely that these associative networks can be associated with the networks representing close relationships. These people become sensitive toward potential signals of rejection and, as a consequence, they might – in a form of "rejection phobia" – avoid initiating or engaging in close relationships in order to avoid being rejected once more.

Treating Social Traumata and Pain With NET
Socially traumatic situations are encoded within sensory-perceptual representations without a solid connection to autobiographical contextual information. For the treatment of these emotions, the same logic applies as to the primary emotions such as fear. The goal of the treatment is to attach the painful emotional responding to the autobiographical context and faciliate a correctional experience through the current close and trusting relationship with the therapist.

Noticeable deviances in interpersonal behavior of the patient, such as mistrust, hiding, withdrawal, or a provocative and verbally aggressive attitude toward the therapist, can be indicators of social abusive experiences. In these cases, the therapist has to be very attentive to biographical events and relationships that relate to rejection, neglect, or degradation. Again, these events must be narrated in detail to embed them in their autobiographical context.

However, there are two major characteristics that challenge the processing of socially aversive events. First of all, social abuses are typically less singular than, e.g., fearful traumatic events, which makes it difficult to focus on a specific event in the narration. However, most patients have outstanding memories of salient prototypical events that represent the provocation of intense shame (Robinaugh & McNally, 2010), emotional abuse, or neglect. To allow the detailed reliving of the emotions that were involved in socially traumatic situations, it is important to concentrate on a few (one to three) of these events rather than reporting a more general and distant version of the abusive story.

The second challenge for narrating social traumata is the fact that the hot memories of interpersonal traumata will ultimately become activated during treatment and may massively interfere with the client–therapist relationship. During moments of high degrees of shame or social pain, the patient may be afraid to be rejected by the therapist. The activation of successive stages of the defense cascade (Figure 1) will provoke an interpersonal stress response, which might result in with-

drawal or verbal aggression toward the therapist. In these cases, it is crucial not to confirm the patient's learned expectations but rather to remain compassionate, empathic, and accepting regardless of the patient's interpersonal behavior. These moments can be a major chance to attach the interpersonal hot memory to the past and to learn that these associations are no longer valid.

It Is Never too Late – 'Mending' Back in Time
The great opportunity during NET is that reactivating an old memory trace renders it vulnerable once again, much as a new memory would be. The stored information about the past is susceptible for change (only) in those very moments, when the associative network is 'hot' again and accessible right during the exposure treatment session. It is as if everything would happen again. The literature shows, that a previously acquired (conditioned) memory can get influenced and disrupted when it is properly reactivated (Nader, Schafe, LeDoux, 2000). In this way the past is indeed present during narrative exposure and can now be changed for the better. For example a person, who revives a recollection of her cold and neglecting mother, can now have an empathic and warm therapist response replacing the former abusive and dismissive parental reaction. In, what we call 'high-end NET', reliving of such past situations of social trauma and experiencing emotional validation within a good therapeutic contact, can mean rescripting the memories and healing the past.

Guilt
Guilt is a common secondary emotion in response to the confrontation with traumatic stressors. Combat exposure, physical abuse, sexual abuse, and the loss of a loved one have all been found to be associated with the experience of trauma-related guilt. Many victims continue to feel guilty about things they have done or not done during the traumatic events. They feel that they have contributed to harm themselves or others. Victims of mass disasters, violence, and wars sometimes feel guilty for having survived, while others who were close to them had to die. Guilt feelings and related ruminations can be extremely disturbing for PTSD patients. In many cases, victims are convinced of their own guilt even if there is no rational reason for this assumption.

Kubany (1994) has suggested different dimensions of guilt in trauma survivors, all of which cause distress:
- Lack of justification for actions taken
- Violation of values or wrongdoing
- Foreseeability and preventability – the degree to which a person thinks she or he knew (in advance)

that a negative outcome was going to occur and could have prevented the outcome
• Responsibility for causing a negative outcome

Victims with high levels of guilt feelings often have a "hindsight bias" about their possibilities to act during the traumatic event. This includes false beliefs that unforeseeable outcomes were foreseeable and therefore preventable and the belief that one was capable of knowing an unforeseeable negative outcome was going to occur and that one could have acted to prevent this outcome. A correction of these wrong appraisals requires correct autobiographical encoding: i.e., a prerequisite for a correct appraisal of what has happened and what the options were is a detailed and autobiographic narration of the event that can challenge guilt on all four dimensions. The narration may give information that in fact the events were much less predictable and preventable than the patient thought, and the responsibility might be shared by many other actors not just the patient. In addition, reliving of their state of mind while they had made a decision that turned out to be wrong later, might help to counteract the hindsight bias and to find justifications for what they have done.

Sometimes it is easier to live with guilt rather than to accept the intense feeling that a person has been completely at the perpetrator's mercy during the traumatic event. In these cases, focusing on the feelings of helplessness in the narration is crucial to help the person to accept this emotion and to embed it into the context of the story. In most cases, much of the reappraisal concerning guilt feelings occurs by itself during the narration. Sometimes it can be useful to spend some minutes after the event to talk about the meaning of it. Let the patient clarify responsibilities and justifications, now that she or he can do it.

3.3.4 The Patient Is Withholding Information

In general, when a patient withholds information from the therapist, or chooses not to disclose certain information, the narration can obviously not proceed. The patient's internal attention is alternatively focused on what is NOT being spoken. Patients often withhold information unintentionally. They feel the information is irrelevant or that the information is too confusing to articulate. Things might cross their mind that they dismiss. They assume it is not important to the work being carried out on the traumatic incident or that it is unrelated. Whether this information is relevant will only be determined if the person dares

to talk freely about all of their experiences they still suffer from.

Here are a few examples of why a patient might withhold information:
• The incident happened early in childhood. The person had no cognitive frame or knowledge base to interpret the meaning of these bodily sensations coming from that time period. The adult still experiences the bodily sensations, but as they were not given meaning at the time, the origin of them is unknown.
• The patient is afraid that the information being shared will get back to somebody else, e.g., the partner.
• It is assumed that the therapist might not understand or not accept what the patient is trying to say.
• Shame, social pain, or guilt prevent the patient from talking about the experiences (see Section 3.3.3).
• The patient feels too much unpleasant arousal, such as a rapid heartbeat, and wants to avoid this feeling.

The therapist might ask any of the following questions to elicit unspoken material:
• „Has anything crossed your mind that you have not mentioned?"
• „Have you thought of something that is difficult to tell me about?"
• „Is there something else you're thinking about right now?"

The patient needs to feel safe enough in the relationship with the therapist to tell her/him whatever crosses her/his mind. If the therapist refrains from judging the patient and from interpreting for the patient, she or he is more likely to feel safe enough to speak frankly. It might be necessary for the therapist to work on safety issues, both exploring the patient's fears and concerns, and providing the reassurance and confidentiality of a good therapeutic alliance.

3.3.5 There Seems to Be No Habituation

At times, it seems as if the narration has progressed nicely, according to the therapist, yet the arousal level of the patient stays high, and habituation has not begun. Usually this is a sign that not all key experiences have been narrated. Something important is missing. Embarrassing or shameful events that have happened may have remained hidden during the first narrative passage through the trauma-related stories. The following are potentially significant issues that a therapist might focus on to detect a missing link.

Here is a checklist for ways to support emotional processing and habituation:

- Check on sensory information contained in the incident. This includes visual images of the incident, somatosensory sensations, olfactory cues (smells), or bodily pains experienced during the incident.
- Focus on what the patient is paying attention to while relating the traumatic event. How much was the patient aware of what was happening in the room? In her own story? In her body? To what extent was she able to pay attention to the sequence of events?
- Check intentions throughout the incident, including conflicting or embarrassing ones.
- Check on actions taken during the incident. Did the patient regret having taken certain actions? Were there actions the patient would have liked to have taken but could not?
- Look for evidence of the patient's cognitions: Thoughts, assumptions, decisions, beliefs, expectations, ideas, and conclusions made during the incident. What did the patient think at the time? What decisions were made? What did she or he believe was going on? What did they think was going to happen next?
- Watch for cognitions: Thoughts, assumptions, decisions, beliefs, expectations, ideas, and conclusions made since the incident. What does the patient believe about her/his condition? What does she/he think will happen to her/him when she/he has a flashback? What are the assumptions she/he has made about why this happened to her/him?
- Look for „mysteries" in the story. Is there information being given that could not have been available to her/him at the time or since then?
- Observe incongruities in the story line. Look for examples of people or things that should have been present at the time or vice versa, but were not. Look for events that should have taken place, but did not. Listen for events that took place, but should not have.
- Check on practical or existential questions that arise from the incident. What does the client feel about the larger meaning of her/his life? What does it mean in terms of her/his day-to-day life?
- Ask about anything the person wanted to communicate but did not or could not during or after the event.
- Ask about anything the person may have found out about herself/himself as a result of the incident.
- Notice strategies that the patient uses to cope with the incident.

In these instances, the therapist carefully forms her or his own questions to enable the patient to assess material that so far has not been forthcoming. The idea is to recover a missing feature of the incident and to incorporate it into the narrative. The following questions are possible examples. They only make sense in the context of the patient's narration:

- "Was there anything you wanted to *say* at the time of the incident but didn't?"
- "Was there anything you wanted to *do* at the time of the incident and didn't?"
- "Were you aware of anything else going on around you at the time of the incident while you were trying to ...?"
- "Did this experience, at the time of the incident, raise questions for you?"
- "You didn't mention any feelings when you talked about this situation.... Were you experiencing any emotions at the time of the incident?"
- "Did you promise anything to yourself or others at the time of the incident?"
- "How did you react when the man said that at the time of the incident?"

Summary

Over time, and with each review of the story, the narrative should be improving in terms of content, focus, and defragmentation. The narrative should be more comprehensive, complete, detailed, and insightful. The person's level of arousal should be calmer over time. If this is true, there is no need for the therapist to interfere with questions. Commonly, however, the therapist needs to assist in improving defragmentation by putting the pieces of the memory-puzzle together. The therapist should be helping to structure the reported elements in time and space.

3.3.6 Therapist Avoidance

Therapists should be aware of the behavior they might employ unwillingly to protect themselves from the horror they are listening to. The therapist might build up resistance as a defense mechanism, or might overly identify with and feel sorry for the patient. The first is called joining the *fraternity of nonbelievers*. This happens when one does not want to shatter one's own deeply rooted beliefs that humans are beings who are inherently good or that the world is a safe place. Listening to the survivor's narrative about the cruelty of perpetrators contradicts these beliefs. The second trap is called the *pitfall of sorrow*. This pitfall involves the therapist feeling more sympathy then empathy for the person's emotions. Other authors have stated that denial is a common way for mental health and relief workers to cope with the problems confronted, to reduce cognitive dissonance, and to preserve self-esteem.

De Waal (1988) proposed two forms of denial. The first form of denial involves the therapist's rejection of responsibility. The mental health or relief worker consciously decides not to take responsibility for the suffering of people or for the effectiveness and result of the treatment interventions. As in major natural disasters, viewing each of hundreds of thousands of people as individuals would paralyze even the most balanced helper (Harrell-Bond, 2002). Just as for the survivors themselves, some manner of coping mechanism is necessary to blunt the truth of this realization. The second form of denial is the helper's tendency to incorrectly rationalize away the truth, convincing oneself, for instance, that refugees from certain cultures would not feel pain and death the way Westerners do, but would be used to death and suffering. The misconception that traumatic events are not disturbing to refugees can lead to a general dehumanization of refugees (Waldron, 1987). Harrell-Bond (1986) commented on this excuse, saying that there is perhaps no more dramatic way of expressing psychological distance or denying a common humanity.

Of course, the patient does not benefit from these defense mechanisms employed by the therapist. Survivors are likely to feel emotionally rejected by the therapist. Patients quickly realize the inability of the interviewer to cope with the emotionally shocking facts of the traumatic incident. In order to not harm, overwhelm, or appall the therapist, victims tend to unconsciously minimize their version to a more socially acceptable story. It is the therapist's responsibility to make sure that she or he realizes her his own mental state and ability to cope. A therapist should receive adequate supervision provided by the team to overcome such mechanisms.

The same is true for the therapist's professional handling of short episodes of emotional outbursts, flashbacks, or brief states of reactive psychosis in the patient. The therapist must not be afraid of such emotions. When painful feelings of the patient find an appropriate way of being expressed in a warm and understanding setting, they will soon come to a natural end. As a rule of thumb, healthy, expressive crying takes about 10-20 minutes. Ongoing toneless, soft whimpering is not productive. The therapist will comfort a person who is crying and will facilitate and support the complete expression of sadness and grief. Expressions of anger should be even shorter, because they are usually covering some underlying pain that will surface next. The patient should be told that as opposed to rage, anger

is a good sign, often a prerequisite of healing. It may thus be important to adequately experience and express anger. It is of inherent importance that the anger is cognitively connected back to the feelings that took place during the traumatic scene.

Note: The therapist should never push or force the patient to experience some kind of catharsis. As a rule, the therapist tries to match the patient's tone and voice, including the melody and frequency level of the patient, and to stay with the client during the narration. When it comes time to wind down, the therapist stays slightly ahead of the patient, leading that process.

Summary   Self-reflection for the therapist

Questions therapists may pose to themselves before beginning trauma-focused work:
- Am I ready to hear this person's story? Might the story be related to my own personal experiences? Will it activate parts of my own fear network?
- What type of support do I need?
- Am I really convinced that it is beneficial for the survivor to be exposed again to the traumatic memories?
- Am I aware of the fact that the survivor probably feels his or her story is incommunicable?
- When and for what do I need peer support, supervision?
- Am I aware of, and how will I handle, the two main pitfalls: (1) maintaining a conspiracy of silence and (2) overly identifying with the patient?

3.3.7 Memory and Reality

On the journey through the life of a patient, it is important for the therapist to keep in mind that *memoire* means reconstruction. The therapist should not expect that the memory of the traumatic events is going to be an exact replication what was seen, heard, or experienced by the person. The therapist should therefore try to imagine the patient's situation at the time of trauma and attempt to understand how the incident is being remembered. The therapist must be particularly aware of the following factors, all of which are known to shape the representation of an event memory (Baddely, 1990; Reviere, 1996; Schacter, 1996):
1. *What were the characteristics of the patient at the time of the event?* How old was the client at the time of the event? What is the gender of the patient? What are the emotional state, physical condition, and circumstances of the patient now and at the time of the event?
2. *What knowledge base did the patient have at the time of the event?* How would the person grasp and

understand what had happened to her/him, her/his family, and to other people? How would she/he have been able to integrate this understanding into the existing background and previous experience?

3. *What is the current interpretation of the events?* How does the patient attempt to make sense of the things that happened? Which aspects of the event does she/he connect to others? How are symptoms that arise from the trauma interpreted?

4. *What retrieval strategies does the patient use, and what is the context of recall?* Which way does the patient try to remember: The objective facts, the individual emotions and physical sensations, or the thoughts at that time? In what condition is the patient now, during the therapeutic encounter with the event? How does she/he currently feel? What characterizes the therapist's contact with her/him? Does the patient feel safe, anxious, sad?

Memory can be affected in many ways. In particular, stress or anxiety alter coding strategies and thus affect accuracy and consistency. Memories change every time they are recalled. During the screening process, the therapist must be aware that certain elements of an event most likely will be fragmentary or incomplete. The joint work of the therapist and patient will be to restore the whole picture, such that it becomes a consistent narration that makes complete sense to the patient.

Sometimes, especially regarding events that happened early in childhood, the patient has intrusive memories but is not sure what happened in the past that created these memory chunks. Some patients wish to recover implicit memories, many of which are presumed to be incidents of childhood sexual abuse. You can agree with the patient to go through the memories with the NET procedure. But make clear to the patient that for childhood events, gaps may remain. The main rule in such a treatment is that the therapist must never be suggestive with regard to what may have happened, and never construct a story that has no clear foundation in the patient's memory. Instead of constructing a false declarative memory (which will then always be in conflict with the implicit knowledge), it is better to help the patient to accept that she/he might be able to recall what exactly has happened.

3.3.8 The Therapist–Patient Relationship: Rules of NET and Standard Ethical Principles

First and foremost, the therapist's role is to facilitate and guide the patient's own testimony process, while maintaining good, empathic contact with the patient in a nonjudgmental way. Here are a few guidelines for this process:

- *The therapist does not interpret for the patient.* The patient is the authority regarding her/his own experience. Therefore, the therapist does not need to agree with the content of what is being said or the way the patient interprets the experiences. The therapist simply agrees to accept it as the patient's truth and world.

- *Therapists do not judge for the patient.* Therapists must not offend, punish, or invalidate the patient or her/his ideas, perceptions, or actions; nor must they praise or validate them. Minor comments, gestures, or facial expressions of the therapist can be a signs of approval or disapproval, which give the impression of judging the patient's actions.

- *Therapists should make sure that they comprehends what the patient is saying.* If not, the patient will feel alone and unsupported. In case of confusion, the therapist must seek clarification by admitting not having understood. The therapist might say, "I did not understand what you said. Could you tell me again?" The therapist will empathically encourage the patient to continue with the story and to express her/his feelings. If the patient should waiver or avoid continuing, it is the therapist's task to encourage the patient to continue narrating in a continuous, linear manner along the timeline of that person's life.

- *Therapists do nothing in a session that counteracts the process of narration.* Therapists do not talk about themselves, make random comments, give lectures, or offer advice. Therapists do not express emotions toward the patient, whether through sighs, signs of anger, anxiety, boredom, or inappropriate laughter. When the therapist stays close to the emotional and cognitive processing of the person, she/he is less likely to perceive details that the patient talks about as disgusting, appalling, intolerable, or shocking. If these feelings do arise, it is not appropriate to show these feelings unscrupulously to the patient. On the contrary, well-considered feedback may be helpful for the survivor, who is usually afraid of what kind of emotions her/his story might evoke in a listener. It is also not therapeutic for patients to feel as if they must take care of the therapist. A professional therapist should seek supervision from colleagues when discomfort arises.

- *Therapists act in predictable ways and with integrity.* This includes educating the patient as to how the NET will proceed, what the therapist will do in a session, and what the expectations will be. Therapists will announce and explain when they need to do something that may be unexpected, such as changing seat positions, getting up from the seat, or moving objects in the room.

- *The therapist will always respect the patient's boundaries.* The therapist should never try to work against a patient's will or in the presence of expressed protest. The therapist has to accept the decision of the patient if they do not want to continue. This does not mean that the therapist has to accept avoidance without further psychoeducation. It is the responsibility of the therapist to inform the patient about the consequences of interrupting treatment and the potential benefits of continuing. A clear decision on the part of a well-informed patient must be accepted. The therapist will always respect an individual's physical need for space. If touching the patient is necessary at any point, get the person's permission, even if you have already discussed the parameters around appropriate touch.

- *The therapist takes complete responsibility for the session, without dominating or overwhelming the survivor.* The therapist will monitor and act in the best interest of the emotional reactions of the patient. To allow the patient to put all of their attention on the testimony process, the therapist, similar to a personal secretary or manager who keeps record of the session, keeps the agenda straight and reminds the patient when she/he needs to take the next step. However, allow the patient to take the action. The therapist must ensure that the session is being given in a suitable space and time; and that the environment is as safe, private, quiet, and comfortable as possible in any given situation. Care should be taken not to interrupt a session for any reason. In case of some external interruption, protect your patient from any harm or threat, or from being seen and identified.

- *The therapist must not transfer care to another therapist without preparation.* In some cases, it might be necessary to transfer the care to another therapist. In this case, inform the patient as soon as possible that this will be happening. Build in a transitional period, if possible, during which the new therapist will join you for a joint session. Allow for cotherapy to take place long enough for a secure bond to form between the patient and the new therapist. The

original therapist will lead the session unless there is some other agreement with the new therapist and the patient. If these steps are not taken, the patient may feel a sense of powerlessness and a lack of control or predictability. Even worse, the patient may feel rejected. The therapist must ensure an environment in which the patient is able to complete the NET procedure successfully.

- *The therapist assures fidelity and confidentiality.* The patient must be absolutely assured that all the information exchanged during the conversation will be treated in a confidential manner. Any written notes will be used only to help reconstruct the experience and to create the written document. The final description will be handed to the patient during the final session. It is then the patient's choice whether this document should be destroyed or preserved and to what extent it should be distributed.

- *The therapist assures the patient that the working relationship will be cooperative.* Tell your patient that you are willing to accompany them in the journey through their life history. There will be no hierarchy, as there might be in some cultures and with certain types of faith healing, such as witchcraft. There will be no healing without mutual cooperation.

- *The therapist is explicit in her/his behavior.* The therapist should inform the patient that there is no such thing as a hidden agenda or manipulative techniques involved. Whatever happens in the sessions will be explained and made explicit beforehand and at any point during the session, if requested.

- *The therapist is responsible for the interpreter.* In many cases, interpreters are necessary. Interpreters must be very well trained (Ruf, Schauer, & Elbert, 2009). The interpreter is bound to all contractual agreements between the patient and the therapist, including confidentiality and ethical principles. The ideal interpreter does not have a "mind of her/his own," but acts as a voice only. The interpreter will need supervision and professional support from the therapist, since interpreters are often from the same ethnic group as the patient and might have had similar experiences as the patient. Interpreters who present with symptoms of traumatic stress must not be employed for translation work.

Appendix

Appendix A: Informed Consent Form

Appendix B: vivo Event Checklist for War, Detention, and Torture Experiences

Appendix C: Modified Adverse Childhood Experience (MACE) Scale (Version 0.9)

Appendix D: Examples of Narrations of Life Experiences Resulting from NET

Appendix E: vivo and Contact Addresses of the Authors

Informed Consent Form

Participant's name: _____

Age: _____   Date of examination: _____

Place of examination: _____

Project title: _____

Project investigators: _____

Explanation of Procedures
I understand that I am being asked to participate in a research study that will explore the effectiveness of therapeutic interventions for reducing symptoms caused by extremely stressful experiences. The treatment approach is called Narrative Exposure Therapy and will require me to create a detailed report of my biography, including traumatic events. With the support of the therapist, I will try to clarify my memories about the traumatic experiences. There will be up to six therapy sessions once or twice a week that will each last around 60-120 minutes. In order to see how helpful this assistance might be, there will be an examination of my symptoms 3 months after the therapy, after 6 months, and after 1 year.

Risks and Discomforts
I understand that in the course of the treatment, the recollections of the traumatic events will be encouraged and may cause personal stress. I understand that the recollections of events that have caused great personal stress may evoke feelings of anxiety and frustration.

Benefits
I understand that the benefits I will receive from participation in this study include free examinations and treatments that may reduce the intensity and frequency of symptoms that arose from extremely stressful experiences. Participation in this study does not imply any financial benefits.

Confidentiality
I understand that information gathered during this study will be kept strictly confidential. I agree that the results may be published for scientific purposes, provided my identity is not revealed and cannot be reconstructed on the basis of the published data.

Withdrawal Without Prejudice and Termination
I understand that I am free to withdraw my consent and to discontinue my participation in this project at any time without prejudice against future care. I also understand that my participation in this study may be ended without my consent, if it is determined by the investigators that it is in my best interest or if I significantly fail to follow study procedures.

Costs to Subject from Participation and Payment and Research-Related Injuries
I understand that there will be no costs for my participation in this study. All examinations and treatments associated with the project will be free; vivo has made no provision for financial compensation in the case of physical or psychological injury resulting from this research.

Legal Rights
I will receive a copy of this informed consent. I am not waiving any of my legal rights by signing this consent form. My signature indicates that I agree to participate in this study.

Agreement
My signature indicates that I have decided to participate, that I have read (or had read to me) the information provided above, and that I have received a copy of this consent form.

_____   _____
Signature of patient (& caretaker in the case of children)   **Signature of therapist**

_____
Signature of witness

From: M. Schauer, F. Neuner, & T. Elbert: *Narrative Exposure Therapy: A Treatment for Traumatic Stress Disorders*   © 2011 Hogrefe Publishing

vivo Event Checklist for War, Detention, and Torture Experiences

This event checklist should only be used in diagnostic interviews by experienced therapists. The interviewer should instruct the patient to remain focused on responding in the affirmative or negative to each item. To minimize their discomfort, patients should not elaborate about the details of their experience at this time. The interviewer should use the following example to address this with the patient prior to the interview:

I am going to read to you a list of several events related to war, detention, and maltreatment. We have collected these situations from other survivors of organized violence who had to undergo fright, abuse, and torture. You might have witnessed or experienced some of these events; others will not apply to you. To minimize your distress during the interview, I am going to read out the listed experiences, and you need only answer whether you have experienced something like that or not. In case I need more details on certain experiences, I am going to ask you very specific questions, which you are free to answer or not. Since it is not necessary to give details of your worst memories, we will attempt to minimize your distress during the interview.

(The interviewer should be familiar with each question before the start of the interview.)

0 Detention/Arrest?	❑ yes / ❑ no
If no: organized violence?	❑ yes / ❑ no
In which city / town was (were) the prison(s)?	
In which year(s) was (were) the imprisonment(s)?	
1 Were you insulted by officials?	❑ yes / ❑ no
2 Beating / kicking wounds/bruises/scars (still visible today?)	❑ yes / ❑ no (❑ yes / ❑ no)
a) Head	❑ yes / ❑ no
b) Body	❑ yes / ❑ no
c) Sole of feet (Falaka)	❑ yes / ❑ no
d) Genital area	❑ yes / ❑ no
Was your head injured?	
– never	❑ yes / ❑ no
– beaten on head/face without visible scars	❑ yes / ❑ no
– Suspected diagnosis of head injury (scars) or craniocerebral injury (unconsciousness)	❑ yes / ❑ no
– Unconsciousness after head injury for (max. time) _____ minutes	
3 Were you blindfolded?	❑ yes / ❑ no
In which situation(s)?	
4 Were you alternately treated very gently and very rudely or even cruelly? (Did your torturers assume different roles?)	❑ yes / ❑ no (❑ yes / ❑ no)
5 Were you forced to stand in a painful position for a long period of time?	❑ yes / ❑ no
Can you describe this position to me?	
6 Were you threatened with (further) torture?	❑ yes / ❑ no
7 Were you prevented from personal hygiene such as daily washing?	❑ yes / ❑ no
8 Was your hair pulled or yanked?	❑ yes / ❑ no
9 Did you receive electric shocks?	❑ yes / ❑ no
On which part of the body? (Where were the electrodes placed?)	
10 Did you have to witness how others were tortured? (relatives, friends, strangers?)	❑ yes / ❑ no
Could you overhear how others were tortured (screams etc.)? (relatives, friends, strangers?)	❑ yes / ❑ no
11 Were you forced to maltreat/torture fellow prisoners?	❑ yes / ❑ no
12 Did anyone threaten to kill you?	❑ yes / ❑ no

From: M. Schauer, F. Neuner, & T. Elbert: *Narrative Exposure Therapy: A Treatment for Traumatic Stress Disorders*   © 2011 Hogrefe Publishing

13	Did you have to take off all your clothes?	❑ yes / ❑ no
	(in which situation(s)?)	
14	Were you prevented from using the toilet when you needed to? (Were you prevented from going for such a long time that you had to urinate in your prison cell and were consequently punished?)	❑ yes / ❑ no
	Did you have to urinate or defecate out of pure anxiety and terror?	❑ yes / ❑ no
15	Were you isolated from other people and fellow prisoners for several days?	❑ yes / ❑ no
	(For approximately how long? In which prison(s)?)	
16	Were you prevented from sleeping regularly?	❑ yes / ❑ no
	(By which means? Were you deliberately deprived of sleep in order to wear you out?)	
17	Were you put in a cell or box that was so small or crowded that you could not move?	❑ yes / ❑ no
18	Were you refused medical assistance when you needed it?	❑ yes / ❑ no
19	Were you exposed to extreme heat or cold?	❑ yes / ❑ no
	What kind?	
20	Were you threatened with violence to your family?	❑ yes / ❑ no
21	Did you have too little to eat for several days (in prison or in a hiding place) so that you had to starve?	❑ yes / ❑ no
22	Did they hang you from a rope or chain (e.g., on the wrists)?	❑ yes / ❑ no
23	Did you receive too little or only dirty water for a long time?	❑ yes / ❑ no
24	Were you hosed down with ice-cold water or did you have to shower with cold water until it hurt?	❑ yes / ❑ no
25	Mock execution: Did your torturers behave as if they were about to kill you?	❑ yes / ❑ no
26	Were you strangled or in another way prevented from breathing (e.g., with a plastic bag)?	❑ yes / ❑ no
27	Did you have to experience *water boarding*? Were you dunked into water or other liquids (e.g., feces)?	❑ yes / ❑ no
28	Were you tied up (for several hours) or affixed in another way?	❑ yes / ❑ no
	(To which object were you tied? How?)	
29	Were you threatened with rape?	❑ yes / ❑ no
30	Were your genitals touched against your will?	❑ yes / ❑ no
31	Were you forced to sexual intercourse against your will or were objects inserted into your anus or genitals?	❑ yes / ❑ no
	(Was this done by several people?)	(❑ yes / ❑ no)
32	Were your arms, legs, or your body (over)stretched by force?	❑ yes / ❑ no
33	Were your genitals (testicles, penis, nipples, etc.) twisted or squeezed?	❑ yes / ❑ no
	Outside prison	
34	Were you ever in the immediate vicinity of armed fighting or shelling/bombing?	❑ yes / ❑ no
35	Did you have to hide from snipers?	❑ yes / ❑ no
36	Were you locked in your house for several days, or did you have to hide in your house?	❑ yes / ❑ no
37	Did you witness other people being sexually abused?	❑ yes / ❑ no
38	Did you witness a member of your family being hurt or killed?	❑ yes / ❑ no
39	Did you ever witness another person being injured or even killed?	❑ yes / ❑ no
40	Did you see mutilations or dead bodies? (People killed by force, grotesquely disfigured bodies of dead people, etc.)	❑ yes / ❑ no

From: M. Schauer, F. Neuner, & T. Elbert: *Narrative Exposure Therapy: A Treatment for Traumatic Stress Disorders*   © 2011 Hogrefe Publishing

41	Were you forced to have any form of contact with blood or dead bodies?	❏ yes / ❏ no
42	Did you witness a person close to you being abducted or arrested?	❏ yes / ❏ no
43	Was your house searched by force by officials or did you experience anything similar?	❏ yes / ❏ no
44	Did you witness collective punishment (witness or victim)?	❏ yes / ❏ no
45	Other experiences? (Did you experience any other extremely frightening event, or was something extremely terrifying done to you, e.g., a so-far-unmentioned method to torment you, or did you experience something extremely unpleasant that we did not list above?)	❏ yes / ❏ no
	– During imprisonment (e.g. torture with snakes, stubbing out cigarettes on the body)	❏ yes / ❏ no
	– Outside imprisonment	❏ yes / ❏ no

Modified Adverse Childhood Experience (MACE) Scale (Version 0.9)

(inspired by the ACE scale; composed by Martin H. Teicher, McLean Hospital/Harvard Medical School & Angelika Parigger, University of Konstanz, used with permission)

Sometimes parents, stepparents or other adults living in the house do hurtful things. If this happened during your childhood (first 18 years of your life) please provide your best estimate of your age at the time(s) of occurrence.
Please check all ages that apply.

For example item 1. Swore at you, called you names, said insulting things like your "fat", "ugly", "stupid", etc. more than a few times a year.
If at ages 6-8 your father swore at you and at ages 8-10 your mother insulted you, and at age 17 your mother's new live-in boyfriend called you names; you would check off as follows:

● Yes ○ No

1	2	3	4	5	6	7	8	9	10	11	12	13	14	15	16	17	18
					✓	✓	✓	✓	✓							✓	

1. Swore at you, called you names, said insulting things like your "fat", "ugly", "stupid", etc. more than a few times a year.
Please check all ages that apply.

○ Yes ○ No

1	2	3	4	5	6	7	8	9	10	11	12	13	14	15	16	17	18

2. Said hurtful things that made you feel bad, embarrassed or humiliated more than a few times a year.
Please check all ages that apply.

○ Yes ○ No

1	2	3	4	5	6	7	8	9	10	11	12	13	14	15	16	17	18

3. Yelled or screamed at you more than a few times per year.
Please check all ages that apply.

○ Yes ○ No

1	2	3	4	5	6	7	8	9	10	11	12	13	14	15	16	17	18

4. Acted in a way that made you afraid that you might be physically hurt.
Please check all ages that apply.

○ Yes_1 ○ No_0

1	2	3	4	5	6	7	8	9	10	11	12	13	14	15	16	17	18

Please indicate if this made you feel helpless or terrified.

❏ Helpless ❏ Terrified

5. Acted in a way that made you afraid that you might be physically hurt.
Please check all ages that apply.

○ Yes_1 ○ No_0

1	2	3	4	5	6	7	8	9	10	11	12	13	14	15	16	17	18

Please indicate if this made you feel helpless or terrified.

❏ Helpless ❏ Terrified

6. Locked you in a closet, attic, basement or garage.
Please check all ages that apply.

○ Yes_1 ○ No_0

1	2	3	4	5	6	7	8	9	10	11	12	13	14	15	16	17	18

Please indicate if this made you feel helpless or terrified.

❏ Helpless ❏ Terrified

From: M. Schauer, F. Neuner, & T. Elbert: *Narrative Exposure Therapy: A Treatment for Traumatic Stress Disorders* © 2011 Hogrefe Publishing

7. Intentionally pushed, grabbed, shoved, slapped, pinched, punched or kicked you.
Please check all ages that apply.

Yes $_1$ ◯   No $_0$ ◯

1	2	3	4	5	6	7	8	9	10	11	12	13	14	15	16	17	18

Please indicate if this made you feel helpless or terrified.

❏ Helpless   ❏ Terrified

8. Hit you so hard that it left marks for more than a few minutes.
Please check all ages that apply.

Yes $_1$ ◯   No $_0$ ◯

1	2	3	4	5	6	7	8	9	10	11	12	13	14	15	16	17	18

Please indicate if this made you feel helpless or terrified.

❏ Helpless   ❏ Terrified

9. Hit you so hard, or intentionally harmed you in some way, that you received or should have received medical attention.
Please check all ages that apply.

Yes $_1$ ◯   No $_0$ ◯

1	2	3	4	5	6	7	8	9	10	11	12	13	14	15	16	17	18

Please indicate if this made you feel helpless or terrified.

❏ Helpless   ❏ Terrified

10. Spanked you with their open hand on your buttocks, arms or legs.
Please check all ages that apply.

Yes $_1$ ◯   No $_0$ ◯

1	2	3	4	5	6	7	8	9	10	11	12	13	14	15	16	17	18

Please indicate if this made you feel helpless or terrified.

❏ Helpless   ❏ Terrified

11. Spanked you on your bare (unclothed) buttocks.
Please check all ages that apply.

Yes $_1$ ◯   No $_0$ ◯

1	2	3	4	5	6	7	8	9	10	11	12	13	14	15	16	17	18

Please indicate if this made you feel helpless or terrified.

❏ Helpless   ❏ Terrified

12. Spanked you with an object such as a strap, belt, brush, paddle, rod, etc.
Please check all ages that apply.

Yes $_1$ ◯   No $_0$ ◯

1	2	3	4	5	6	7	8	9	10	11	12	13	14	15	16	17	18

Please indicate if this made you feel helpless or terrified.

❏ Helpless   ❏ Terrified

13. Made inappropriate sexual comments or suggestions to you.
Please check all ages that apply.

Yes $_1$ ◯   No $_0$ ◯

1	2	3	4	5	6	7	8	9	10	11	12	13	14	15	16	17	18

Please indicate if this made you feel helpless or terrified.

❏ Helpless   ❏ Terrified

14. Touched or fondled your body in a sexual way.
Please check all ages that apply.

Yes $_1$ ◯   No $_0$ ◯

1	2	3	4	5	6	7	8	9	10	11	12	13	14	15	16	17	18

Please indicate if this made you feel helpless or terrified.

❏ Helpless   ❏ Terrified

15. Had you touch their body in a sexual way.
Please check all ages that apply.

1	2	3	4	5	6	7	8	9	10	11	12	13	14	15	16	17	18

Please indicate if this made you feel helpless or terrified.

Yes₁ ○ No₀ ○
Helpless ❑ Terrified ❑

16. Attempted to have any type of sexual intercourse (oral, anal or vaginal) with you.
Please check all ages that apply.

1	2	3	4	5	6	7	8	9	10	11	12	13	14	15	16	17	18

Please indicate if this made you feel helpless or terrified.

Yes₁ ○ No₀ ○
Helpless ❑ Terrified ❑

17. Actually had any type of sexual intercourse (oral, anal or vaginal) with you.
Please check all ages that apply.

1	2	3	4	5	6	7	8	9	10	11	12	13	14	15	16	17	18

Please indicate if this made you feel helpless or terrified.

Yes₁ ○ No₀ ○
Helpless ❑ Terrified ❑

Sometimes parents, stepparents or other adults living in the house do hurtful things to your siblings (brother, sister, stepsiblings).
If this happened during your childhood (first 18 years of your life) please provide your best estimates of your age at the time(s) of occurrence.
Please check all ages that apply.

18. Intentionally pushed, grabbed, shoved, slapped, pinched, punched, or kicked your sibling (stepsibling).
Please check all ages that apply.

1	2	3	4	5	6	7	8	9	10	11	12	13	14	15	16	17	18

Please indicate if this made you feel helpless or terrified.

Yes₁ ○ No₀ ○
Helpless ❑ Terrified ❑

19. Hit your sibling (stepsibling) so hard that it left marks for more than a few minutes.
Please check all ages that apply.

1	2	3	4	5	6	7	8	9	10	11	12	13	14	15	16	17	18

Please indicate if this made you feel helpless or terrified.

Yes₁ ○ No₀ ○
Helpless ❑ Terrified ❑

20. Hit your sibling (stepsibling) so hard, or intentionally harmed him/her in some way, that he/she received or should have received medical attention.
Please check all ages that apply.

1	2	3	4	5	6	7	8	9	10	11	12	13	14	15	16	17	18

Please indicate if this made you feel helpless or terrified.

Yes₁ ○ No₀ ○
Helpless ❑ Terrified ❑

21. Made inappropriate sexual comments or suggestions to your sibling (stepsibling).
Please check all ages that apply.

1	2	3	4	5	6	7	8	9	10	11	12	13	14	15	16	17	18

Please indicate if this made you feel helpless or terrified.

Yes₁ ○ No₀ ○
Helpless ❑ Terrified ❑

22. Touched or fondled your sibling (stepsibling) in a sexual way.
Please check all ages that apply.

1	2	3	4	5	6	7	8	9	10	11	12	13	14	15	16	17	18

Please indicate if this made you feel helpless or terrified.

Yes$_1$ ○   No$_0$ ○
Helpless ❑   Terrified ❑

23. Had your sibling (stepsibling) touch their body in a sexual way.
Please check all ages that apply.

1	2	3	4	5	6	7	8	9	10	11	12	13	14	15	16	17	18

Please indicate if this made you feel helpless or terrified.

Yes$_1$ ○   No$_0$ ○
Helpless ❑   Terrified ❑

24. Had or attempted to have any type of sexual intercourse (oral, anal or vaginal) with your sibling (stepsibling).
Please check all ages that apply.

1	2	3	4	5	6	7	8	9	10	11	12	13	14	15	16	17	18

Please indicate if this made you feel helpless or terrified.

Yes$_1$ ○   No$_0$ ○
Helpless ❑   Terrified ❑

25. Threatened to harm your sibling (stepsibling).
Please check all ages that apply.

1	2	3	4	5	6	7	8	9	10	11	12	13	14	15	16	17	18

Please indicate if this made you feel helpless or terrified.

Yes$_1$ ○   No$_0$ ○
Helpless ❑   Terrified ❑

Sometimes adults or older individuals NOT living in the house do hurtful things to you. If this happened during your childhood (first 18 years of your life) please provide your best estimates of your age at the time(s) of occurrence.

Please check all ages that apply.

26. Made inappropriate sexual comments or suggestions to you.
Please check all ages that apply.

1	2	3	4	5	6	7	8	9	10	11	12	13	14	15	16	17	18

Please indicate if this made you feel helpless or terrified.

Yes$_1$ ○   No$_0$ ○
Helpless ❑   Terrified ❑

27. Touched or fondled your body in a sexual way.
Please check all ages that apply.

1	2	3	4	5	6	7	8	9	10	11	12	13	14	15	16	17	18

Please indicate if this made you feel helpless or terrified.

Yes$_1$ ○   No$_0$ ○
Helpless ❑   Terrified ❑

28. Had you touch their body in a sexual way.
Please check all ages that apply.

1	2	3	4	5	6	7	8	9	10	11	12	13	14	15	16	17	18

Please indicate if this made you feel helpless or terrified.

Yes$_1$ ○   No$_0$ ○
Helpless ❑   Terrified ❑

29. Attempted to have any type of sexual intercourse (oral, anal or vaginal) with you.
Please check all ages that apply.

○ Yes₁ ○ No₀

1	2	3	4	5	6	7	8	9	10	11	12	13	14	15	16	17	18

Please indicate if this made you feel helpless or terrified.

❑ Helpless ❑ Terrified

---

30. Actually had sexual intercourse (oral, anal or vaginal) with you.
Please check all ages that apply.

○ Yes₁ ○ No₀

1	2	3	4	5	6	7	8	9	10	11	12	13	14	15	16	17	18

Please indicate if this made you feel helpless or terrified.

❑ Helpless ❑ Terrified

**Sometimes intense arguments or physical fights occur between parents, stepparents or other adults (boyfriends, girlfriends, grandparents) living in the household.
If this happened during your childhood (first 18 years of your life) please provide your best estimates of your age at the time(s) of occurrence.
Please check all ages that apply.**

---

31. Witnessed adults living in the household argue intensely with your mother (stepmother, grand-mother), say derogatory things to her, or threaten her with harm.
Please check all ages that apply.

○ Yes₁ ○ No₀

1	2	3	4	5	6	7	8	9	10	11	12	13	14	15	16	17	18

Please indicate if this made you feel helpless or terrified.

❑ Helpless ❑ Terrified

---

32. Witnessed adults living in the household argue intensely with your father (stepfather, grandfa-ther), say derogatory things to him, or threaten him with harm.
Please check all ages that apply.

○ Yes₁ ○ No₀

1	2	3	4	5	6	7	8	9	10	11	12	13	14	15	16	17	18

Please indicate if this made you feel helpless or terrified.

❑ Helpless ❑ Terrified

---

33. Saw adults living in the household push, grab, slap or throw something at your mother (step-mother, grandmother).
Please check all ages that apply.

○ Yes₁ ○ No₀

1	2	3	4	5	6	7	8	9	10	11	12	13	14	15	16	17	18

Please indicate if this made you feel helpless or terrified.

❑ Helpless ❑ Terrified

---

34. Saw adults living in the household hit your mother (stepmother, grandmother) so hard that it left marks for more than a few minutes.
Please check all ages that apply.

○ Yes₁ ○ No₀

1	2	3	4	5	6	7	8	9	10	11	12	13	14	15	16	17	18

Please indicate if this made you feel helpless or terrified.

❑ Helpless ❑ Terrified

| 35. Saw adults living in the household hit your mother (stepmother, grandmother) so hard, or intentionally harm her in some way, that she received or should have received medical attention. Please check all ages that apply. | | | | | | | | | | | | | | | | | | Yes $_1$ ◯   No $_0$ ◯ |

1	2	3	4	5	6	7	8	9	10	11	12	13	14	15	16	17	18

Please indicate if this made you feel helpless or terrified.   ❏ Helpless   ❏ Terrified

---

36. Saw adults living in the household push, grab, slap or throw something at your father (stepfather, grandfather).
Please check all ages that apply.   Yes $_1$ ◯   No $_0$ ◯

1	2	3	4	5	6	7	8	9	10	11	12	13	14	15	16	17	18

Please indicate if this made you feel helpless or terrified.   ❏ Helpless   ❏ Terrified

---

37. Saw adults living in the household hit your father (stepfather, grandfather) so hard that it left marks for more than a few minutes.
Please check all ages that apply.   Yes $_1$ ◯   No $_0$ ◯

1	2	3	4	5	6	7	8	9	10	11	12	13	14	15	16	17	18

Please indicate if this made you feel helpless or terrified.   ❏ Helpless   ❏ Terrified

---

38. Saw adults living in the household hit your father (stepfather, grandfather) so hard, or intentionally harm him in some way, that he received or should have received medical attention.
Please check all ages that apply.   Yes $_1$ ◯   No $_0$ ◯

1	2	3	4	5	6	7	8	9	10	11	12	13	14	15	16	17	18

Please indicate if this made you feel helpless or terrified.   ❏ Helpless   ❏ Terrified

---

Sometimes children your own age or older do hurtful things like bully or harass you. If this happened during your childhood (first 18 years of your life) please provide your best estimates of your age at the time(s) of occurrence.
Please check all ages that apply.

---

39. Swore at you, called you names, said insulting things like your "fat", "ugly", "stupid", etc. more than a few times a year.
Please check all ages that apply.   Yes $_1$ ◯   No $_0$ ◯

1	2	3	4	5	6	7	8	9	10	11	12	13	14	15	16	17	18

Please indicate ages when (if) the person doing this to you was a date (e.g., boyfriend, girlfriend, someone you associated with on a social, romantic or intimate level).   Yes $_1$ ◯   No $_0$ ◯

1	2	3	4	5	6	7	8	9	10	11	12	13	14	15	16	17	18

---

40. Said hurtful things that made you feel bad, embarrassed or humiliated more than a few times a year.
Please check all ages that apply.   Yes $_1$ ◯   No $_0$ ◯

1	2	3	4	5	6	7	8	9	10	11	12	13	14	15	16	17	18

Please indicate ages when (if) the person doing this to you was a date.   Yes $_1$ ◯   No $_0$ ◯

1	2	3	4	5	6	7	8	9	10	11	12	13	14	15	16	17	18

41. Said things behind your back, posted derogatory messages about you, or spread rumors about you.

◯ Yes₁ ◯ No₀

Please check all ages that apply.

1	2	3	4	5	6	7	8	9	10	11	12	13	14	15	16	17	18

Please indicate ages when (if) the person doing this to you was a date.

◯ Yes₁ ◯ No₀

1	2	3	4	5	6	7	8	9	10	11	12	13	14	15	16	17	18

42. Intentionally excluded you from activities or groups.

◯ Yes₁ ◯ No₀

Please check all ages that apply.

1	2	3	4	5	6	7	8	9	10	11	12	13	14	15	16	17	18

Please indicate ages when (if) the person doing this to you was a date.

◯ Yes₁ ◯ No₀

1	2	3	4	5	6	7	8	9	10	11	12	13	14	15	16	17	18

43. Acted in a way that made you afraid that you might be physically hurt.

◯ Yes₁ ◯ No₀

Please check all ages that apply.

1	2	3	4	5	6	7	8	9	10	11	12	13	14	15	16	17	18

Please indicate ages when (if) the person doing this to you was a date.

◯ Yes₁ ◯ No₀

1	2	3	4	5	6	7	8	9	10	11	12	13	14	15	16	17	18

44. Threatened you in order to take your money or possessions.

◯ Yes₁ ◯ No₀

Please check all ages that apply.

1	2	3	4	5	6	7	8	9	10	11	12	13	14	15	16	17	18

Please indicate ages when (if) the person doing this to you was a date.

◯ Yes₁ ◯ No₀

1	2	3	4	5	6	7	8	9	10	11	12	13	14	15	16	17	18

45. Forced or threatened you to do things that you did not want to do.

◯ Yes₁ ◯ No₀

Please check all ages that apply.

1	2	3	4	5	6	7	8	9	10	11	12	13	14	15	16	17	18

If yes, please describe examples:

Please indicate ages when (if) the person doing this to you was a date.

◯ Yes₁ ◯ No₀

1	2	3	4	5	6	7	8	9	10	11	12	13	14	15	16	17	18

46. Intentionally pushed, grabbed, shoved, slapped, pinched, punched, or kicked you.
Please check all ages that apply.

Yes₁ ○   No₀ ○

1	2	3	4	5	6	7	8	9	10	11	12	13	14	15	16	17	18

Please indicate ages when (if) the person doing this to you was a date.

Yes₁ ○   No₀ ○

1	2	3	4	5	6	7	8	9	10	11	12	13	14	15	16	17	18

47. Hit you so hard that it left marks for more than a few minutes.
Please check all ages that apply.

Yes₁ ○   No₀ ○

1	2	3	4	5	6	7	8	9	10	11	12	13	14	15	16	17	18

Please indicate ages when (if) the person doing this to you was a date.

Yes₁ ○   No₀ ○

1	2	3	4	5	6	7	8	9	10	11	12	13	14	15	16	17	18

48. Hit you so hard, or intentionally harmed you in some way, that you received or should have received medical attention.
Please check all ages that apply.

Yes₁ ○   No₀ ○

1	2	3	4	5	6	7	8	9	10	11	12	13	14	15	16	17	18

Please indicate ages when (if) the person doing this to you was a date.

Yes₁ ○   No₀ ○

1	2	3	4	5	6	7	8	9	10	11	12	13	14	15	16	17	18

49. Forced you to engage in sexual activity against your will.
Please check all ages that apply.

Yes₁ ○   No₀ ○

1	2	3	4	5	6	7	8	9	10	11	12	13	14	15	16	17	18

Please indicate ages when (if) the person doing this to you was a date.

Yes₁ ○   No₀ ○

1	2	3	4	5	6	7	8	9	10	11	12	13	14	15	16	17	18

50. Forced you to do things sexually that you did not want to do.
Please check all ages that apply.

Yes₁ ○   No₀ ○

1	2	3	4	5	6	7	8	9	10	11	12	13	14	15	16	17	18

Please indicate ages when (if) the person doing this to you was a date.

Yes₁ ○   No₀ ○

1	2	3	4	5	6	7	8	9	10	11	12	13	14	15	16	17	18

From: M. Schauer, F. Neuner, & T. Elbert: *Narrative Exposure Therapy: A Treatment for Traumatic Stress Disorders*   © 2011 Hogrefe Publishing

Please indicate if the following happened during your childhood (first 18 years of your life). Please provide your best estimates of your age at the time(s) of occurrence.
Please check all ages that apply.

51. You felt that your mother or other important maternal figure was present in the household but emotionally unavailable to you for a variety of reasons like drugs, alcohol, workaholic, having an affair, heedlessly pursuing their own goals.
Please check all ages that apply.

○ Yes$_1$ ○ No$_0$

1	2	3	4	5	6	7	8	9	10	11	12	13	14	15	16	17	18

52. You felt that your father or other important paternal figure was present in the household but emotionally unavailable to you for a variety of reasons like drugs, alcohol, workaholic, having an affair, heedlessly pursuing their own goals.
Please check all ages that apply.

○ Yes$_1$ ○ No$_0$

1	2	3	4	5	6	7	8	9	10	11	12	13	14	15	16	17	18

53. You felt that your mother or other important maternal figure was emotionally unavailable to you for a variety of reasons like military service, taking care of a sick relative, in school, business necessity.
Please check all ages that apply.

○ Yes$_1$ ○ No$_0$

1	2	3	4	5	6	7	8	9	10	11	12	13	14	15	16	17	18

54. You felt that your father or other important paternal figure was emotionally unavailable to you for a variety of reasons like military service, taking care of a sick relative, in school, business necessity.
Please check all ages that apply.

○ Yes$_1$ ○ No$_0$

1	2	3	4	5	6	7	8	9	10	11	12	13	14	15	16	17	18

55. A parent or other important parental figure was very difficult to please.
Please check all ages that apply.

○ Yes$_1$ ○ No$_0$

1	2	3	4	5	6	7	8	9	10	11	12	13	14	15	16	17	18

56. A parent or other important parental figure did not have the time or interest to talk to you.
Please check all ages that apply.

○ Yes$_1$ ○ No$_0$

1	2	3	4	5	6	7	8	9	10	11	12	13	14	15	16	17	18

57. One or more individuals in your family made you feel loved.
Please check all ages that apply.

○ Yes$_1$ ○ No$_0$

1	2	3	4	5	6	7	8	9	10	11	12	13	14	15	16	17	18

Who? (e.g. mother, aunt, maternal grandfather)

58. One or more individuals in your family helped you feel important or special.
Please check all ages that apply.

1	2	3	4	5	6	7	8	9	10	11	12	13	14	15	16	17	18

Yes$_1$ No$_0$

Who? (e.g. mother, aunt, maternal grandfather)

59. One or more individuals in your family were there to take care of you and protect you.
Please check all ages that apply.

1	2	3	4	5	6	7	8	9	10	11	12	13	14	15	16	17	18

Yes$_1$ No$_0$

Who? (e.g. mother, aunt, maternal grandfather)

60. One or more individuals in your family were there to take you to the doctor or Emergency Room if the need ever arose.
Please check all ages that apply.

1	2	3	4	5	6	7	8	9	10	11	12	13	14	15	16	17	18

Yes$_1$ No$_0$

Who? (e.g. mother, aunt, maternal grandfather)

61. One or more individuals in your family would help you with your homework, or to get ready for school.
Please check all ages that apply.

1	2	3	4	5	6	7	8	9	10	11	12	13	14	15	16	17	18

Yes$_1$ No$_0$

Please indicate if the following statements were true about you and your family during your childhood, and your age at the time(s) you felt this to be true.
Please check all ages that apply.

62. You didn't have enough to eat.
Please check all ages that apply.

1	2	3	4	5	6	7	8	9	10	11	12	13	14	15	16	17	18

Yes$_1$ No$_0$

63. You had to wear dirty clothes.
Please check all ages that apply.

1	2	3	4	5	6	7	8	9	10	11	12	13	14	15	16	17	18

Yes$_1$ No$_0$

64. You were left unsupervised at an age or in situations when you should have been supervised.
Please check all ages that apply.

1	2	3	4	5	6	7	8	9	10	11	12	13	14	15	16	17	18

Yes$_1$ No$_0$

65. You felt that you had to shoulder adult responsibilities.
Please check all ages that apply.

1	2	3	4	5	6	7	8	9	10	11	12	13	14	15	16	17	18

Yes$_1$ No$_0$

66. You felt that your family was under severe financial pressure. Please check all ages that apply.																			Yes $_1$ ◯	No $_0$ ◯
1	2	3	4	5	6	7	8	9	10	11	12	13	14	15	16	17	18			

67. One or more individuals kept important secrets or facts from you. Please check all ages that apply.																			Yes $_1$ ◯	No $_0$ ◯
1	2	3	4	5	6	7	8	9	10	11	12	13	14	15	16	17	18			

68. Your parents were separated. Please check all ages that apply.																			Yes $_1$ ◯	No $_0$ ◯
1	2	3	4	5	6	7	8	9	10	11	12	13	14	15	16	17	18			

69. Your parents were divorced. Please check all ages that apply.																			Yes $_1$ ◯	No $_0$ ◯
1	2	3	4	5	6	7	8	9	10	11	12	13	14	15	16	17	18			

70. A parent or other important parental figure died. Please check all ages that apply.																			Yes $_1$ ◯	No $_0$ ◯
1	2	3	4	5	6	7	8	9	10	11	12	13	14	15	16	17	18			

71. You had to spend time living in two or more households. Please check all ages that apply.																			Yes $_1$ ◯	No $_0$ ◯
1	2	3	4	5	6	7	8	9	10	11	12	13	14	15	16	17	18			

72. You lived in foster care. Please check all ages that apply.																			Yes $_1$ ◯	No $_0$ ◯
1	2	3	4	5	6	7	8	9	10	11	12	13	14	15	16	17	18			

73. People in your family looked out for each other. Please check all ages that apply.																			Yes $_1$ ◯	No $_0$ ◯
1	2	3	4	5	6	7	8	9	10	11	12	13	14	15	16	17	18			

74. People in your family felt close to each other. Please check all ages that apply.																			Yes $_1$ ◯	No $_0$ ◯
1	2	3	4	5	6	7	8	9	10	11	12	13	14	15	16	17	18			

75. Your family was a source of strength and support. Please check all ages that apply.																			Yes $_1$ ◯	No $_0$ ◯
1	2	3	4	5	6	7	8	9	10	11	12	13	14	15	16	17	18			

Examples of Narrations of Life Experiences Resulting from NET

(All original names and places have been changed)

Narrative exposure therapy (NET), by Thomas Elbert & Patient Onyut

I was born on March 23, 1976, in South-West Province, Mundemba, Cameroon. My family is originally from Kribi, South Cameroon; however, my dad established his business in Mundemba. There were four children in my family: I have three younger brothers. We were a very good and happy family. I was the oldest son, so I had many rights and could get whatever I wanted from my father. I started school and completed primary school in South West Province. I did well in secondary school and intended to study politics.

While in school, I started having problems with my chemistry teacher, Fanzo. He was a member of CPDM, the ruling party, which had been in power since February 2, 1982. During the parliamentary elections we were to have a chemistry test. Fanzo promised that if the ruling party were to win the election, there would be an extra percentage mark in the test for every student. However, the opposition party won the election, but power was given to the ruling party. I would have passed my chemistry test, but Fanzo failed me because I stood up against the ruling party. I didn't take it too hard. After failing the test, I was affirmed in my political beliefs.

At that time, I used to show off a lot in school because my dad was a member of the opposition party. I would get punished in school, for example by being given a large area to clean or by being suspended. Suspension from school used to hurt me the most.

When I was 18 years old, I organized a rally with other children that went on for 2 weeks. After school, I put my school uniform in my backpack and headed to the rally with my gang. In those days if they found you demonstrating in uniform they would make you clean the streets. We were made to remove old cars and other obstacles that the demonstrators had used to block the street to cut off the police. The street was full of policemen and opposition party members. The rally went well and I came back home safely.

I formed another gang of children and demonstrated against the illegitimate elections. We used to make petrol bombs in response to them shooting and killing my friends. These bombs could not kill – only injure. This was one of the ideas I came up with. Many times they also shot at me but missed.

I was 18 years old when I started politics. My father told me that no matter how I did at school, if I stood up for my rights, I would be a great man in the future. So I became more active. My father was an important member of the SDF Party in the South West. While my father was still alive, I used to go to demonstrations with other students. I was always on the front line. Sometimes I was taken to prison for a couple of hours and beaten. They would tell me to quit my political activities. During some of these incidents, I thought that I was going to die. This happened a few times before my father died.

During one incident I was taken to prison for hours and beaten. This happened as follows: After a demonstration, I was driving in a car. At a checkpoint, the police asked for my driver's license. After recognizing my name, they ordered me to turn on my lights. They ordered me to do other things and asked me questions that annoyed me, and I became angry. They asked me to give them my identity card but I refused. We had a verbal quarrel. One of them slapped me. I told him not to slap me again, or I would slap him back. (In my country, we do not talk back to officers.) We began to fight. They started beating me with their batons. I kept quiet, and they stopped beating me and handcuffed me. They drove to the police station with my car. They took me straight to a room and chained me to a chair, without even writing a statement or anything. They put electrodes to my temples for about 1 second. I screamed. They put them on again. They tortured me for a couple of seconds and let me go only after several hours. I felt okay the next day and went on with my work. I still feel pain in my head sometimes, though. My father brought this case to court, but it was not taken seriously.

The worst case before my father died happened in 1995. I still have a mark on my body – it's a long mark on my back. We used to make campaigns before the elections. During one demonstration, I was together with very good political friends of mine. As students, we used to sing in the streets. I was the leader of the group. My friends and I were caught together as we were running away. We tried to escape into the adjacent streets, but we were surrounded. We ran into the policemen that were ahead of us. They scattered the group with teargas. When I was caught I was beaten. I saw what they did to a friend of mine. His feet were swept out from underneath him. He fell down. Then they kicked him with their boots. It was very sunny and hot on that day. They turned his face and smashed it into the hot concrete. When he lifted his head, it looked like his face was burnt. I was still being beaten. I cried as I watched him, because I was afraid the same thing would happen to me. I was very afraid that I would be the next. (I have a headache now as I talk about it, my hands are cold, my veins stand out, and my is heart beating fast right now.) We were taken to the police station separately. I was released the next day. This was the worst case before my father died because of what they did to my friend, which also could have happened to me. Sometimes I imagine what I would look like now, if the same thing had happened to me.

One day, life became very hard. They burnt down my father's shop. I saw it; I was at home. It was 6.00 AM and we were sleeping. We heard people shouting: "Fire!" and I could smell it because the fire was very big; the sky was red everywhere. I jumped out of my bed and ran outside. My dad, mom and younger brothers followed. There were a lot of people outside. I discovered that it was my father's shop that was on fire. I was struggling with an axe to break the wall with the valuable things behind it, but it was too late. I went inside the building. I was very nervous and angry during the incident. I was in the very middle of it. I could have even burnt to death in there. I did not think of anything while I was inside, or that I could die; I just thought of saving everything. There was a tarpaulin high up that came down and fell behind me. That is how I hurt my thumbnail. It was all black. (I even showed it to the people in Genf. This one here is a new nail, which has just grown.) We did not manage to save anything from the fire. Apart from the goods, my father had also kept some money in the store. Luckily, no one was hurt in the fire. The ruling party had started the fire. My father had no other investments. Life became a little bit harder for us, but I continued going to school.

When I think about it now I become nervous immediately. Not fearful, but angry. I feel like fighting or harming someone, the bad people or the ruling party. I am afraid only when there are many of them, and I am alone. I feel very bad – angry and sad about the fire and because of what we lost.

One day, my father left the house to meet some friends to discuss political issues. It was at around 5:30 or 6:00 in the evening. Our house was very big so either my father or I could leave the house without the other noticing. But, in this case I knew he had left the house. On his way back, he was killed. I was at home. I received a phone call 3 hours after he had left saying that he had died. The caller simply said: "Your father's body is lying in the street beside his car." I went there in one of our other cars. I was not driving; someone else drove. All I saw was my dad's body lying by his car. One side of the car door was open, as if he had been struggling to get out of the car. He had been shot in the heart. Blood was coming out. I rushed to him to see if I could save him. When I reached him I touched him, but his body was already cold. I saw the blood and the bullet in his chest. The bullet was still in his body. Some other people, friends and Party members, came and helped me to bring him to the mortuary because there was nothing else to do. His body stayed in the mortuary for 2 weeks. Then he was given a burial.

Just after my dad died, I could not hold myself back anymore, and I truly went crazy. My family members locked me up to try to calm me down. One friend took me to his own family, 10 kilometers away. He kept me there for some days. A lot of people came to see me there and to arrange the burial because back then I was not able to do anything. The opposition members helped me to arrange the burial. They did most of the organizing and consulted me because I was the oldest son.

It was a big burial because my dad was well known in Cameroon. Even some ministers attended it. He was buried in Kribi. He had only been a visitor in Mundemba. We kept a wake till 11 PM, then we travelled all the way to Kribi from 11 PM till 6 AM the next day. The roads were bad and we were very tired. The chiefs were informed, and they all came to the burial. He was buried the next day at 4.00 PM.

I stayed in Kribi for a week after that; then I went back to Mundemba. My mother came with me, and then she returned to Kribi after a few weeks. She had to go back to the village to mourn her husband, and only came home during the weekends. We mourned my father wearing only white. I was ill after the death of my father. I had a fever for a couple of weeks, and I had a lot of headaches. (I have a headache now as I talk about it. I started having these headaches – not when I saw his dead body – but at the moment I got the news of his death.) I was on relaxants for some time in order to recover quickly. Some friends came to keep us company in our house in Mundemba.

Life became very tough, and still is today, because now I was the head of the family. The day my father died, I did not really feel in danger because I knew they had got what they wanted. Actually I was in more danger before he died because I had been the son of an important opposition party member, and they could get to him by getting me. After his death, I actually became an active member of the Party and that put my life in danger again.

I feel angry because of the death of my dad. He was not sick. We never got to say goodbye. I lost more than a father; I also lost a leader and an ideal. I remember all the good things he did for me. After his death, I no longer felt safe. I knew that I could be killed as well. Others had been killed before my father – he was not the first. I knew some of them, and there were others who I had not known.

Sometimes I see my dad in my dreams. I see him how he was when things were still good and he was still alive. I never see him dead; I only see how he was when life was good. When I see other people's parents of the same calibre as my dad, I feel bad because I have no one to call my own daddy or mum. No one can feel good in such a situation. I shed a lot of tears.

Nobody could help me now with school, and I had to stop my education. I feel angry because my father's good friends, people he used to eat and drink with and discuss issues with (for example, the Assistant Inspector of Police, and the General Manager of the CDC), did not show up to help us after he died.

When I dropped out of school, I became a full-fledged member of the SDF (Social Democratic Front). They gave me a post as a propaganda secretary. I used to publish and distribute fliers whenever there was a rally or a meeting. One day, when I was doing this, a policeman came up to me and asked me why I chose to do these things. He said that maybe this was why my life would end. He talked to me politely while I was putting up the fliers. I said that until the President stepped down, I would continue my political work.

Some time after my father died, presidential elections were held. The President went around campaigning. We were demonstrating in the streets. Schools were closed. We began making petrol bombs again.

One day, when we went out to demonstrate, we were on our way to meet another group in order to attack the military together. There were over 150,000 demonstrators. My best friend was next to me on the front line. Some of the demonstrators had bombs and flags. Even important Party members were there. The policemen were in front of us, facing us. They commanded us to stop and disperse, but we continued to march. They shot teargas at us. They shot it inside the group. We started to fight against them; we threw petrol bombs and stones and anything that could hurt them. They shot real bullets at us – real bullets, not rubber ones. We were shocked. These people were so evil, so evil. My friend and I were carrying a lot of bombs, which we distributed to others to fire them. Suddenly we saw a helicopter. It started to throw teargas at us. We started running, each one for himself. Ahead of us the policemen were already waiting. Gendarmes, policemen, and the military surrounded us. We were running to a hospital that was 1 kilometer away; we wanted to hide there. We found the military already there. We were shocked to see that they were beating people who were inside the hospital. (I feel very angry as I remember this). My friends and I turned around. The helicopter, which was not just from Mundemba or Duala but had come all the way from Yaounde, had landed and dropped off some soldiers. My friend was shot in the foot by one of them. He fell down. I shouted his name. He shouted back. I tried to help him but I couldn't. There was a crowd of soldiers coming towards us. They were still shooting, and the teargas was too much: I had to run to save my own life. My friend was killed and his corpse was left there. I did not actually see how he died. (It was very painful for me, I feel very angry. I do not feel guilty because I did all I could and I had to save my own life).

I was not at home for 3 days, because I was well-known. I knew one of the men who had shot at us. We went to his house when nobody was there. We broke the door open. We set a fire and burnt his military uniform, his video machine, and all the important things that he had. Then we ran away. I felt happy and satisfied that we did this, because it paid for my friend's death. I was happy to do even more. This incident happened about 1 month after the death of my dad.

There was a military celebration on the 1st of June 2000, about 3 months after the death of my dad. After my dad had been killed, I was the next target. On the night of the 31st of May, I was assigned to distribute pamphlets. These pamphlets said that we needed freedom of speech and human rights in our country. I finished the job before midnight and returned home. The rally was to be in Bertoua, in the morning of June 1st, though it would be celebrated in all of Cameroon. But the President would be in Bertoua in the East. We planned to block the streets.

At midnight, there was a knock on my door. At that time, I used to have my own room, away from my family's house, for security. Sometimes I would sleep in my room, and sometimes I slept at home. I was surprised to hear the knock. I went to open the door, but it was broken in before I reached it. When I was still about 3 meters away from the door, I was confronted with about six policemen. The policemen came in and started to hit me everywhere on my body. They wore blue uniforms with black berets. I struggled and fought with them. They hit me on the forehead with the butt of a gun and my forehead broke open. Blood started running down my face, and into my mouth and eyes. They dislocated my arm and knocked out one of my teeth with the butt of a gun. They made a hole in my arm and blood ran out. I still struggled and fought with them, but they were too many for me. They beat me severely until I was unconscious. I was unconscious for 3 days. After a few days, I realized that I was in a cell. There was blood all around me. Even the other prisoners asked the police why they did not take me to a hospital first before taking me to the prison.

In the prison, they fed us beans that were only have cooked once a day. The toilet was in the cell. Everything was being done in there. We were undressed before we entered the cell. They had caught me as the leader of my group in order to disband my group. Nobody knew that I was there. While in the cell, a policeman told me that many prisoners had passed through their hands and died, and so would I. I replied that I would die fighting for my rights and for human rights.

I could not stand up. My whole body was injured. They did not beat me again, because I had so many injuries; I had wounds all over. I couldn't sleep, and I had no appetite. They did not clean me, and I received no medical care. I was never washed for the whole time that I was in the cell. I had no power left even after I had recovered.

I was in the cell until the 17th of July. On that day a policeman asked me where my family lived so that they could be informed where I was. I replied that I would rather die alone than together with my family. He left and only came back on the night of the 18th, because they were working in shifts. He was a just man, but he was working for the government and had to obey their rules. He came to my cell at midnight and removed the chain from my feet. I did not know what was happening. I had had no contact with my family. No one knew where I was, so no one had visited me. The policeman asked me to walk out into the night. That's what they usually did to get rid of people: They asked you to walk into the forest or an open place and shot you from behind. He told me to go and not look behind. I knew this was the end of my life. I thought of my mum and my younger brothers. I started thinking about dead people and where they were, and what the place was like where they were. There was a car ahead of me with four people in it, blinking its lights at me. Two of the people were in uniform, and the other two weren't. When I tried to pass the car, they said, "Come here!" I was shocked. The policeman was now no longer behind me. They handed me a pair of trousers and put me into the car. I sat in the back, in the middle seat. I recognized one man from my village Kribi. The commissioner, with four stars, sat in the front. They drove me from Limbe to Duala. That is a 2-hour drive. When we arrived, they cleaned all the blood off my body. I did not know what was happening. I was surprised to see a policeman being nice to me. In the morning they gave me bread and tea.

At night I was taken to the international airport. The man from my community told me that I had to leave the country for my own safety. If I were to remain in Cameroon, I would die. He told me that they had planned to put me in raw acid the next week. No one checked me at Duala Airport, because the Commissioner was ahead of me escorting me. I didn't have a passport. At the entrance of the plane, a man beside me gave me a passport with my photograph on it but not my name. It was checked at the airport under a mercury bulb, but it was okay. I was checked normally as I boarded the plane. I asked the man if he could tell me who he was, but he said that I had no right to know. I came into Switzerland wearing the slippers I had been wearing in the cell. I had been tortured in them, and I had to hold them together with a pin now.

We left the country at 11:55 and the plane landed in Vienna at 6:30. There we transferred and took a Swiss Air plane to Zürich. This was the last time I saw the man. He took the passport off me. He gave me 40 DM, shook my hand, and said that he had hereby completed his job. He told me to go a human rights organization. He advised me to go to Genf.

It was my first time in Europe. I was afraid of the police, even though they were White. I took the next train to Genf, where I was interviewed 3 days later. Since then, I have had no contact with my family. Sometimes when

I see Black people I become suspicious of them. I know I am not safe yet. I saw my name on the Internet, declared "wanted." I never went online again. I believe that even now there are still people looking for me. If the opposition party comes into power, I might go back to Cameroon. But if I go back to Cameroon now, it will be the end of my life.

Excerpt from a narrative exposure therapy (NET), by Maggie Schauer

Lifeline of Roza Magomadov

I was born on June 28, 1956. I was born into a good family. I had three sisters and five brothers. We were living in a village in Kazakhstan.

I had a good time at school. I had a math teacher who had a big influence on me, and a couple of good friends.

I had an accident and injured my spine.

After having finished 10th grade (in Russia, schooling ends after 10th grade) we moved to Grozny. In Grozny, I started studying educational science and went to a teacher training college for 4 years. At the college, I met my former boyfriend who was studying with me. He was the love of my life, and the time with him was the happiest time period of my life.

When I was 21 years old and in the last year of my studies, my boyfriend died in a car accident.

I started an apprenticeship as a commercial assistant. I liked the training very much and when I started to work in this field I enjoyed it a lot.

My wedding and happiness with my husband, Ali.

Birth of my first son (1985), Alex.

Birth of my second son (1987), Umar. I had a normal life until the war started in 1990.

From 1990 until 2000, we went through a very hard time. The riots in Grozny started in 1990. My grandmother on my mother's side died.

In 1993, they threw a hand grenade in the house of my mother's brother, and his wife died immediately while he died from his injuries a bit later. That year, I witnessed the death of a young man, and one day our car was shot at while we were driving.

1994/1995 First Chechen War. We were evacuated and our family was separated. Later I learned that my husband had died. I never found out what happened to my son. For 4 or 5 years we were constantly on the run.

April 1996 (Grozny): At the beginning of the war, I was beaten and sexually abused. Umar was not with me when it happened. Later we fled to another town.

Early 1998: I witnessed a massacre: About 200 women who had gone to fetch water were shot.

Winter 1999: We made an attempt to escape to Ingushetia, but the car that was supposed to pick us up never arrived. In the same year, they found my mother-in-law, but she was so confused that she was not able to tell me what had happened with my son.

In 2001: Umar and I arrived in Germany.

2004: Officials wanted to deport us: The police came for us at night and we had to spend one night in prison.

2006: Death of my father: A grenade exploded while he was praying.

2007: Death of my mother: She had a heart attack when she heard that I had been raped. At first she was paralyzed and then she died.

September 2006: My son qualifies for university admission. We are happy in Germany for now, but I am still afraid that we will be deported.

My wishes for the future:
1. I would like Umar to obtain a university degree
2. I hope that Alex will be found
3. I wish for my son and myself that we can stay here until the end of our life, that we can feel safe and that my son will find his future here
4. For myself, I am wishing for health

My name is Roza Magomadov and I was born on June 28, 1956 into a good family; unlike most other men, my father neither drank nor smoked. We were living in a village in Kazakhstan. I had three sisters and five brothers, and I was the third child of our parents. Altogether, my mother gave birth to twelve children, but three of them died.

We had a happy life in our village. We did not have a lot of money since my father was the only one in our family who was working, but we were a happy family (*it makes me smile, when I think back, it is a nice feeling to remember this*). My brother Malik and I used to play a lot together. For him I was the older sister who was looking after him, particularly at school. Malik was a very good-natured child; he never had any problems with our parents or with other children. (*These memories make me sad and make me cry as he's dead. At home I can't grieve because my son Umar doesn't know that he is dead*).

......

After having finished 10th grade (in Russia, schooling ends with 10th grade), we moved to Grozny.

......

One day, something terrible happened: It was in Grozny, around the end of April or the beginning of May in 1996. The snow had already melted, but it was not warm yet. We lived in a half-destroyed house in the city of Grozny. Once again, this was a temporary solution. It was very cold; I remember that we stacked pieces of wood for making fire on the concrete floor. There were some mattresses and a couple of blankets, and there were many other women with their children. Plastic bags, not window grates, were covering the windows. These bags were white. One could constantly hear shots from the street; sporadically during the day and a lot during the night. Actually, at that time there was a ceasefire, but nevertheless there were shootings; we could hear the gunshots and see the flashes. I was scared and there was a constant feeling of unrest inside me, the feeling that I should run away. (*Right now I can see the whitish light shine through the bags into the room from the right*). There was a room that was a bit warmer for the children. We were about 15 women while the men were in another part of the house. We used to cook for them, and some Chechen men provided us with food and water. The constant threat of war had been around for a long time now, and for a long time we had not had a home. Our mood was accordingly. In Chechnya we say: "Moving house three times is almost as bad as a house burning down," and all we did in this war was move around. Our life was a catastrophe: It was very very hard, and we all had been tired and demoralized for a long time.

It was always dusky in these ruins, and on the day that I am going to talk about it was almost dark outside. It was after lunch, and the children were in the adjoining room which could be heated, when a couple of Russian soldiers arrived. We could not lock the door because they had broken the lock and used to come and go as they pleased. They entered the house without knocking. They came in order to "check." We did not know any of these men, but I realized at once that they were drunk as they had a smelly alcohol breath; they were cursing a lot. They knew what they wanted; the one who had come in first said straightaway: "Our boss said that we are supposed to have fun here." I assumed that they were hungry and wanted us to make them some food, as we would usually make food for these Russian fools. But they did not want to eat, they said: "We are all now going to chose one of you and fuck you *(trachat)!*" We women were actually not that young anymore as the youngest among us were 35-years-old. I was around 40. These soldiers were younger than us! They all had weapons: Each of them had a Kalashnikov. All the women were together in one room, and a lot of men entered. We were sitting on the floor and leaning against the wall. After they had announced what they wanted, we got scared and starting talking to each other. One of them grabbed a woman called Mila. I was still hoping that the men had meant that she was supposed to work for them, like cook for them or do the washing. We were screaming and wanted to do something! But then one man said to another man: "Akhmed, this one's yours." When I heard that, I understood. He added: "When you're finished with her, it will be my turn."

With this sentence, all my hope was gone, and I was overwhelmed by great weakness. I could not sit up any longer; I was like a wash rag. It was so humiliating (*strong feeling of helplessness*). The woman was next to me on a mattress on the floor. She did not start screaming straight away since she first tried to defend herself. He pushed her with his hand, and she fell. When we saw this crudeness, our apprehension became inescapable certainty. (*Pain in the neck; touches her neck with her hand*). The men surrounded the screaming women while I and a couple of other women went to Mila in order to help her. I wanted to release her from the grip of this man. While I was fighting, I felt strong rage, and I felt the urge to hit him with something, like a stone. I looked around but there was nothing I could have used. *(I can see his pig-face right now!)* It is hard to believe but he even looked quite nice and harmless, around 22 years old and well-built…. This contradiction was sickening somehow. We could have been his mothers. I kept looking for an object but could not find anything when suddenly I was hit from behind: A man hit me with his gun on the right shoulder. I started panicking! He pulled my hands back, held my wrists behind my back and twisted them. Now I was completely helpless and in terrible pain. He dragged me out of the room. There were no doors to the main room, just a blanket that was hanging in the door frame.

He pushed me to the room where Mila was and then they dragged us through several rooms till we reached the back part of the ruin. It was dark and wet. He ripped off my clothes; I was wearing a light coat and its buttons came open straightaway. I felt terribly ashamed and was in a state of total panic. He was very brutal and greedy: He wanted to have me straight away! At once! He was already half-undressed and became angry when it took a while until he managed to pull down my nylon tights. He cursed and threatened me and swore in Russian: "You battered whore!" *(disgust and anger).* He tried to kiss me, but I squirmed and turned my head away. His hands were everywhere: On my breasts and then also in my vagina. *(Hears her own screams.)* He looked "evil." He had light hair and blue eyes. He said: "You are not the first, you Chechen women all have to go 'through us.'" He was very close to me, and I could feel his body heat. I hated his hands on my body, and I hated having to feel his body. Everything inside me was struggling. He smelt of alcohol and sweat, like a man smells when he has not taken care of himself for a while. His sour bad breath like cold smoke was mixed with his body odor. *(Waves of revulsion go through my body, I am literally shaking with disgust.)* He threw me on a wooden pallet, as if I was just an object. He was brutal like an animal, as if he wanted to destroy me. I was lying on my back, and he forcibly penetrated my vagina with his penis. Straightaway I felt a strong pain *(hate and desperation).* He pushed his penis hard inside me several times, and then he came on me, on my face. He was kneeling next to my head and wanted to push his penis into my mouth while I was fighting; trying to press my mouth shut and turn my head away as much as possible *(strong disgust).* There was such a bad smell. *(Turns her head away and shivers.)* And then suddenly I scratched his face in blind fury: I wanted to rip out his eye and I wanted him to be blind on this eye! I wanted him to remember! He kept trying to push his penis into my mouth while shouting at me angrily. Then I opened my mouth a bit and bit into his penis as strongly as I could. I do not know how badly I managed to hurt him, but he went crazy: He screamed with pain and hit me in the face so brutally that I blacked out and fainted.

When I regained consciousness, I was in a "med-point" in a dilapidated house which served as a kind of military hospital. I do not remember how I got there, but when I woke up I immediately remembered what had happened and I was very ashamed….

KIDNET, by vivo international team Elisabeth Schauer, Verena Ertl, & Siyad Bulle, 2003

I was born in M., Somalia, in 1990. I have no brothers and sisters. The house of my family was a few miles outside of town. It was a big house, and we had a good life. My father was a businessman; he owned a shop. My mother stayed at home. Later I was told that both parents were very happy to have me, since they had waited a long time for a child. I didn't know that. I only felt their love. There are some occasions that I remember clearly: when I was 5 years old we celebrated my birthday with a party at our home. I was very happy then. Later, when I was 6 years old I was taken to school. I was very good at school. I remember that I got a special degree. I was the best in my class. My family and I were very happy and proud because of that. I even remember the date of this special day; it was the 15th of August. During the coming school break, my father took me on a trip around the country to reward me. When we came back we met my mother again at home. My mother bought new clothes for me, and I got many presents, like video games. It was the time of the Idd festival. I had my friends at school. I invited them home. We played together. My father took us out to nice places, like the beach. When I remember this, I wished this life would come back, I was very happy then. When I was 9, my father took me to a city called N. for the first time. We were staying in my aunt's home; she used to live there. My aunt was "cool as ice"; she liked to be with kids a lot. She also introduced me to other relatives there. She held a big party for me at her place. However, I remember missing my mother a lot. At least we had phone contact during our trip. I was looking forward to going back home to M. But when we came back, the city was in chaos. Fighting was going on. We heard that my mother had to flee the town. I was crying heavily and regretting having left. But my father calmed me down and assured me that we would be together with my mother soon. I did not know at the time that I would never see my mother again. We have not found her until today.

Shorty after our return then, I went to the market with the house girl. We wanted to buy some new shoes for me. She was inside a shop. I stood in the street, attracted by shoes in a shop window. Suddenly I heard bullets; there was shooting and panic in the street everywhere around me. People were shouting and running. I can hear the sound of the bullets right now when I remember this, some people were shouting: "Allah Aq'bar," and there was the sound of bullets: "drrrrumm, drrrumm, drrrrumm." I fell down and was crouching close to the ground in the street with my hands over my head to protect myself. A moment later I could feel people running over me. I can feel the pain of their feet on my back right now, how they were stepping on me. My heart is beating fast when I remember this, there is a pain in my back and chest. My head is hurting so much right now. I was injured and in that moment I thought I would die. I started crying. The house girl must have recognized my voice; she heard me crying. She had been hiding under a roof, and when she heard me she ran towards me. She was injured too and crying. She wore only one shoe and was bleeding from her head and mouth. She picked me up from the ground and carried me in her arms. I felt I was safe with her. Her name was Amina, she was about 19 or 20 years old then and very beautiful. She called a taxi, we sat inside and drove away. We were safe in this car, and we held each other tightly. I had slung my arms around her, and she had her arms closely around me. We were both crying. There was still shooting, running and people crying around us in the street, but I felt safe. As we went out of the city, the bullets became fewer. We reached home. My father was there. He held me and hugged me. In that moment all pain was gone, I forgot about all my injuries. All I felt was "I am safe now." My father took Amina and me to the hospital. We were treated in the same room, lying on beds next to each other. People were there with aid kits. I had terrible pain in my chest. I was bleeding a lot from the nose. I was coughing blood. I still get the nose bleed now when I remember this day. I also get the pain in my chest, and my heart beats fast whenever I remember. I stayed in the hospital for 2 weeks. Then it was time to say goodbye to Amina, I thought we would part only for a few weeks. We sat together for about 30 minutes and said goodbye to each other. When I remember that moment I feel happy and sad at the same time. Happy because she was the best housekeeper I ever had. She was like a sister to me; she cared for me so much. She saved me, even though she had been scared and injured herself. Since that day I have never seen her again. That makes me very sad every time I think of it.

When I came out of hospital I was somehow ok, but still feeling very low. My father took me to my grandma. She was living in a village further away from M. He thought it would be safer for us there. The village was called K. and was not far from the ocean. In K. I made several good friends after some time. I went to Madaras Qu'ran school again.

About 1 month after I had moved to the village, I walked around with some friends. By that time the war had nearly reached the village. I wanted to look at the ocean because I liked looking at the water a lot. It always made me calm and happy. My friends went into the forest, so we separated. I went to the ocean alone. When I got to the shore, I stood on a rock and looked down over the water. What I saw was horrible. The water was full of dead bodies up to my feet. At first I had thought people were out swimming. But I realized that there were about 20 floating bodies. They were black, there was blood, most of them were children, about 8 or 9 years old, some women, even pregnant ones with big bellies and a few men. The bodies were floating there with their faces up and the eyes wide open. Their stomachs were already swelling. The moment I saw all these dead bodies I got a shock. I started shouting and crying: "Woowooowoo..!" I was shaking all over, I was frozen there on the rock although all I wanted to do was to run away. I felt intense fear, my heart was racing. I even feel it now, when I talk about this moment.

My friends heard me and came. They took me home. The memory of the street shooting in M. had also come back strongly. My nose started bleeding, I had a terrible headache, and the pain in my back where people had stepped on me came back badly. At home, I got first aid, my father put a piece of cloth on my head and neck. For 1 week I could not talk, I could not eat, I was in a state of total shock. Then my grandmother managed to calm me down, she explained about life and death to me, she said: "We all have to die one day; when the time comes that God has decided for you, you will die, no matter if there is war or not, that will be your day...." Slowly the confusion in my head cleared up. I became clearer in my thoughts. I started eating and talking again and felt ok. I woke up from that stage, walked around with my friends again and went to school.

At that time I met Halimo, she was a friend of some of my friends. She had heard about what had happened to me. One day she asked me how I was doing now. This was the first time we talked to each other. She was my age and very beautiful, her skin was dark brown. We liked each other instantly. Soon we were spending most of the time together. We were walking around the neighborhood and talking a lot. When I wanted to go running, she went with me. We went to the shops together, and she helped me with the housework. She taught me a lot of things, and I taught her other things that she did not know. She was like Amina, she cared for me and was kind. We were having a great time. She was so cool. We started giving little gifts to each other. One of them was a postcard that she gave me one day. It read: "Love with all my friendship and all my heart." Halimo was always there for me whatever I wanted to do. She went with me and helped me forget all the bad things that had happened to me. We shared the root of our hearts. Can you ever forget such a beautiful friend?

One day we came back from the Madaras school together. We were a group of about 20 girls and boys. It was about 1:30 PM in the afternoon. We separated because everybody had to walk in different directions to get home. Soon only Halimo and I were left. We decided to use a shortcut. It was a narrow path, bush-land with some trees. We were talking. Suddenly there were 3 grown-up men in front of us. They had guns. Four others showed up behind us. Halimo was the one who realized first that they were killers. She took my left hand, pulled me, and we ran sideways into the bushes. One of them started shooting. It was rapid fire, one bullet hit my buttock, on the left side. At first I didn't feel the pain, then I noticed that my left leg was failing to function. It became awfully heavy. Then the pain came. It was a strong pumping kind of pain. I wanted to get away, so I grabbed my trousers with my hands and tried to pull the leg forward. I had worn white trousers that day. My left side was already full of blood. It was running down my leg, soaking the white cloth. My hands were full of blood, too. Then my leg became too weak. I fell down. Halimo was still pulling my hand. She tried to get me back up, so we could continue running. She was crying and shouting: "Get up, let's run, please! Abdul, let's run!" Her face was full of fear, her eyes were wide open, looking terrified. I couldn't talk; I was just looking at her. One of the men had already reached us and hit me with the back of his gun on the left side of my head from behind. I fainted. I must have been unconscious for about 1 minute. When I woke up I was lying on my stomach, bleeding. I felt the pain in my injured leg. I couldn't see properly. I touched and rubbed my eyes. I thought I would go blind. Everything I saw was red and flickering or flashing, like a red curtain in front of me. And then I saw Halimo, she was about 5 meters away, lying on her back. Two men were holding her arms. All 7 men were there. They were looking ugly; their cloths were dirty and torn. Halimo's clothes were torn, and she was naked. One of the men had pulled down his trousers to his knees. I saw him penetrating her, moving up and down. One side of his face was very damaged. There was hardly any skin, and the left eye was like pushed inside the skull. It was so ugly and disgusting, I was horrified. When I remember this, I start seeing everything red, like in that very moment. When I look at the faces of men in such a state of memory and fear, any face in front of me can turn into the face of that rapist. That's when I lose control. All I want is try to beat and chase the person. I can get very angry and aggressive. It sometimes happens even when it is the face of my father, or other people who I like and admire. Then I feel like as if there are two people inside me. While the deformed man was raping Halimo, the others were standing there watching, laughing, and constantly shooting into the air. These are the only sounds I could hear, and they are ringing in my ear whenever I think of that day. Halimo's lips were swollen and bleeding. She was injured on her right cheek near the eye. Her eyes were open and dark. She seemed to be unconscious. I felt terrible pain. But I tried to move, shout, do anything, throw a stone at least, to make them stop, but I was frozen, paralyzed. I could not move. I was annoyed and very angry. My body failed me completely; I could not move at all. I was trapped. I felt so helpless and guilty. Since then I blame myself for not helping her, whereas she was always helping me so much. This guilt and sadness has weighed very heavy on me ever since. When the first man had finished, the next one was raping her. He was the one with the scar. He pulled off his clothes in a hurry. He wore a long shirt. He was penetrating her, too. When I saw him moving up and down, I fainted again. It was just too much; it was too terrible to bear. The next thing I remember was that I woke up seeing white things. There were voices talking. First I thought I was in another world, or dead, or something like that. I was in hospital. I saw blood dripping from a bottle on the right side of my bed. It was an infusion. My dad was there beside me. He was holding my hand. I was still fearing a lot. Then a doctor came and for the first time the face of an ordinary man turned into the disgusting face of the rapist. I was terrified and screamed: "This is the guy I saw and I know what he did!" I was furious and angry, full of tension. My dad tried to calm me down, but I shouted: "I will kill you!" My dad explained to me that it was just the doctor, and that he wanted to help me. My father also tried to find out what had happened to me, but I could not tell him.

After that incident I got a single room for a period of time. The nights in the hospital were horrible. I couldn't sleep. I saw the face of the rapist. I saw everything red when I remembered. I could not eat. I was blaming myself for what had happened. I was feeling guilty. I was terribly angry. A very deep feeling of darkness came into my heart and has never left me up to today. I had no future, no hope. After some time, when I seemed to have become more normal, it was decided that I should share a room again. But it didn't take long, and I attacked my roommate. I shouted at him and pulled at his infusion because I thought he, too, was one of the rapists. So I was moved to a solitary room again. I was having nightmares about the rape scene and the dead bodies floating at the shore all the time. When I saw children playing and being happy I had to cry because I thought I could never do something like that again. I was in hospital for 3 months. In the end I was somehow okay again. Then the day I left the hospital, at the gate my dad and I met a stranger and again everything turned red and I saw the rapist in that innocent man. I ran after him, shouted at him, and wanted to hurt him. My father got me and held me tight. He said: "What is wrong with you? What's wrong?" I have never told him or anybody else what had happened to me exactly during that day of the rape, and he also doesn't know what goes on in my mind and body when I get out of control. This is why I felt and still feel a certain distance to everybody around me. People don't understand why I act strange sometimes, and I cannot tell them.

Some time later Halimo's parents visited me at my home. They had brought gifts and wanted to see how I was doing. I could not face them. I could not open the door. I felt so bad and guilty. How could she ever forgive me for not having helped her when she needed me most? Sometimes she comes to me in my dreams, even now, and she looks beautiful and kind, just like she used to. But I cannot forgive myself. I don't even know whether she is still alive. I can't get myself to find out. I can't imagine how it would be to see her again. I only know I would run away.

After my days in the hospital my father took me to a friend of his. He lived in a small and quiet village. There were a lot of children in the village, playing football. I spend most of the time inside, just watching them, doing nothing. I was completely absent, far away, dealing with the darkness in my heart. After 3 weeks in the village I started to relax a bit. I ate more and slept a bit. Then fighting reached even this little remote village. One day at 12 noon, there was a heavy attack. There were explosions, fire, and the sounds of bullets all over the place. First, I was inside the house alone. People ran around and fled towards the forest. I was full of fear, shocked and paralyzed, but I ran behind the house. From there I could not move, I just stood there, my heart was racing and my whole body was shaking. Many people were passing by, some were injured, some shot, some were running although they were lacking an arm. One man lying very near to me on the ground was torn into two parts. A shell must have hit him. His upper part was lying far from his lower part, yet he was still crying and screaming. There was a lot of blood. The sight of him was horrible, it just looked so awful. All I did was close my eyes, I could not move. I don't know how long I was frozen there in terror and fear, crying until my dad came and carried me into a pickup. He was holding me as I was shaking and crying. I sat beside my dad and the driver in the front seat. Suddenly, as we were already heading out of the village, a bullet hit our driver through the front window. The glass shattered. The bullet went into the front of his head and something came out of his neck. The driver fell backwards and blood spilled over my eye. The vehicle lost control, and we went into a ditch with great speed. When the pickup crashed,

I was catapulted out through the window and fainted. When I woke up I was lying halfway on the front of the car, halfway on the ground. I was more or less ok and immediately checked on my dad. He was unconscious, blood was coming out of his mouth, and his shoulder and chest were injured. By that time people had come, and they helped us on a truck to get to the nearby hospital. My father was unconscious for a long time. I kept sitting by his bedside, holding his hand and talking to him. I was scared he would not come back. I told him: "Don't worry. I'm ok. Please wake up, wake up!" I stayed in the hospital with my dad for 2 weeks, for there was no other place I could have gone to. Sometimes a guy came and gave me some fruit to eat.

When my dad was feeling better we went to friends and they brought us to G. There we met my aunt. We stayed there for a while. My dad had no job. He was just there with me thinking about what should happen to us in the future. I was feeling safer in G. but I had still problems with sleeping. After a while my aunty married, and I was somehow happy, but there was nothing I could enjoy any more, even the marriage party was not enjoyable for me.

Then we decided to move on to U. In U. I made new friends and one day we met at a friend's place to watch the movie *Black Hawk Down*. It is a film about the war in Somalia. At first it was okay, but when the shooting in the film started and a lot of blood was shown I got out of control. I started to see everything red, I was breathing fast, my heart was racing. I got scared, furious, angry. I started shaking and then I took a chair and threw it into the TV screen. The television exploded and everybody screamed and shouted. I didn't realize the panic and chaos around me. It was like I was not in my world anymore. I was full of panic, I ran out of the room and down the stairs. I fell and cut my tongue badly, blood was dripping out of my mouth and on my trousers. I was still in total shock and panic when they found me. I was taken to hospital and treated for about 1 month. I could not talk properly for some time because my tongue was swollen and stitched together. My dad did not understand what had happened. He just said he had to pay a lot of money for the damage that I had done.

In those days we were living with another aunt, actually it was not my aunt, it was the wife of one of my dad's friends. Altogether we spent about 1 year in U. My dad was unemployed during that time, but he was helping the friends we stayed with.

Then in 1999 my dad got to know a woman from Tanzania in U. They decided to get married, and we moved to the refugee camp in 2000. The woman is okay, although I don't talk to her too much. She also doesn't know anything about my past, and I don't know what she thinks is wrong with me when I get out of control. Sometimes she makes an effort and tries to talk to me. She asks me questions about my experiences in the past, but I cannot tell her. She tries, but still I do not feel very close to her.

Even now, many years later, the pictures of the day when Halimo got raped keep coming back to my mind. I look at normal people, like a teacher or a friend, and suddenly the face of the rapist appears. Then I get angry and aggressive and try to hurt the person. I throw things and get violent. Sometimes I find myself sitting in strange places, like on top of the roof, crying, and I have no idea how I got there. It is as if there are two personalities living inside me. One is smart and kind and normal, the other one is crazy and violent. I try so hard to control this other side of me. But I fail. Sometimes I feel tears running down my cheek, and I wonder why. Sometimes I walk down the street, and suddenly I see the path in the bush of that day in front of me and I feel Halimo's hand pulling my hand, trying to make me run and escape together. Since that day I can't walk shortcuts anymore. Even a normal bush can bring back all these memories. And when the memory of the rape comes, all the other pictures are in my mind as well, like the dead bodies in the ocean. Since we are in the camp it is especially bad, since there is so much bush land around.

Now that I have talked about all that has happened to me, I would also like my father to know. I want him to read my story. I also want to register now with the Red Cross Tracing Service, to find Halimo. Maybe she is still in Somalia or lives as a refugee in Nairobi. Wherever she is now, I want to find out how her life is today. May be she will write to me, or we can even meet? Until today, I have never started a friendship with a girl again. I didn't want to get close to them anymore. They remind me of what happened to Halimo and me. In the future I wish I can live like a normal person, get married, and have children. I would like to be a doctor or a lawyer. I would love to help people.

Date and Place:

_____   _____   _____
Signature Survivor   Signature Therapist   Signature Interpreter

vivo and Contact Addresses of the Authors

Who is vivo
The organization vivo is an alliance of professionals experienced in research and service provision in the fields of psychotraumatology, public health, human rights advocacy, humanitarian aid, behavioral neuroscience, and sustainable development.

The mission of vivo
As an organization, vivo works to overcome and prevent traumatic stress and its consequences within the individual as well as the community, safeguarding the rights and dignity of people affected by violence and conflict. The further aims of vivo are to strengthen local resources for the development of peaceful, human rights–based, societal ways of living.

Program areas of vivo
The organization vivo focuses on traumatic stress in different societal and cultural settings. Scientific research is carried out in the field to systematically learn from the victims themselves and disseminate their knowledge. The organization develops, implements, and evaluates evidence-based best practice interventions. It provides training for local and international professionals who assist those who have fallen victim to psychological trauma and human rights abuse. The organization raises awareness among the general public and decision makers on issues related to trauma and its consequences. It also documents violations of human rights and helps those affected find redress by working with national and international agencies. Scientists, field practitioners, and those affected are brought together by the organization to foster collaboration and partnership building for multidisciplinary trauma and mental health program development.

url: www.vivo.org

Contact addresses of the authors:
Dr. Maggie Schauer, e-mail: maggie.schauer@uni-konstanz.de
and
Prof. Dr. Thomas Elbert, e-mail: thomas.elbert@uni-konstanz.de
are at the vivo Outpatient Clinic and at the University of Konstanz, Dept of Psychology
Postal address:
Centre for Psychiatry, Feursteinstr. 55, Haus 22, D-78479 Reichenau, Germany; fax: +49-7531-88-4623

Prof. Dr. Frank Neuner, e-mail: frank.neuner@uni-bielefeld.de
is at the University of Bielefeld, Dept. of Psychology; Postbox 100131, D-33501 Bielefeld, Germany

References

Agger, I. (1994). *Trauma and testimony among refugee women: A psycho-social exploration.* London: Zed Books.

Agger, I., & Jensen, S. B. (1990). Testimony as ritual and evidence in psychotherapy for political prisoners. *Journal of Traumatic Stress, 3,* 115–130.

Aldenhoff, J. (2009). The challenge psychotherapy (Herausforderung Psychotherapie). *Ärztliche Psychotherapie, 4,*206–216.

American Psychiatric Association. (1994). *Diagnostic and statistical manual of mental disorders* (4ᵗʰ ed.). New York, NY: Author.

American Psychiatric Association. (1997). *Let's talk facts about mental illnesses – An overview.* New York, NY: Author. Retrieved from www.psych.org/public_info/

American Psychiatric Association. (2000). *Diagnostic and statistical manual of mental disorders – DSM-IV-TR* (4th edition, text revision). Washington, DC: American Psychiatric Association.

Amnesty International. (2003). *Definitions of torture.* Retrieved January 7, 2003, from http://www.amnesty.org.uk/torture/definition.shtml

Anda, R. F., Felitti, V. J., Bremner, J. D., Walker, J. D., Whitfield, C., Perry, B. D., Dube, S. R., & Giles, W. H. (2005). The enduring effects of abuse and related adverse experiences in childhood A convergence of evidence from neurobiology and epidemiology. *European Archives of Psychiatry and Clinical Neuroscience, 256,* 174–186.

Andersen, S. L., & Teicher, M. H. (2008). Stress, sensitive periods and maturational events in adolescent depression. *Trends in Neurosciences, 31,* 183–191.

Baddely, A. L. (1990). *Human memory.* Boston, MA: Allyn & Bacon.

Barnett, O. (2001). Why *battered* women do not leave: Part 2: External inhibiting factors, social support and internal inhibiting factors. *Trauma, Violence, and Abuse, 2,* 3–35.

Bauer, P. J. (1996). What do infants recall of their lives? Memory for specific events by one- to two-years-olds. *American Psychologist, 51,* 29–41.

Bettelheim, B. (1986). *Surviving the Holocaust.* London, UK: Fontana.

Bichescu, D., Neuner, F., Schauer, M., & Elbert, T. (2007). Narrative Exposure Therapy of political imprisonment-related chronic trauma-spectrum disorders. *Behaviour Research and Therapy, 45,* 2212–2220.

Bisbey, S., & Bisbey, L. B. (1998). *Brief therapy for post-traumatic stress disorder: Traumatic incident reduction and related techniques.* Chichester, UK: John Wiley & Sons.

Blanchard, E. B., Hickling, E. J., Forneris, C. A., Taylor, A. E., Buckley, T. C., & Loos, W. R., et al. (1997). Prediction of remission of acute posttraumatic stress disorder in motor vehicle accident victims. *Journal of Traumatic Stress, 10,* 215–234.

Bock, J., Helmeke, C., Ovtscharoff, W., Gruß, M., & Braun, K. (2003). Frühkindliche emotionale Erfahrungen beeinflussen die funktionelle Entwicklung des Gehirns. *NeuroForum, 2,* 51–57.

Bohus, M., Limberger, M. F., Ebner, U. W., Glocker, F. X., Schwarz, B., Wernz, M., Lieb, K. (2000). Pain perception during self-reported distress and calmness in patients with borderline personality disorder and self-mutilating behavior. *Psychiatry Res. 95,* 251–260.

Bonne, O., Brandes, D., Gilboa, A., Gomori, J. M., Shenton, M. E., Pitman, R. K., & Shalev, A. Y. (2001). Longitudinal MRI study of hippocampal volume in trauma survivors with PTSD. *American Journal of Psychiatry, 158,* 8.

Bremner, J. D. (2002). *Does stress damage the brain? Understanding trauma-related disorders from a mind-body perspective.* New York, NY: W. W. Norton.

Bremner, J. D., Krystal, J. H., Southwick, S. M., & Charney, D. S. (1995). Functional neuroanatomical correlates of the effects of stress on memory. *Journal of Traumatic Stress, 8,* 527–545.

Bremner, J. D., Randall, P., Vermetten, E., Staib, L., Bronen, R. A., Mazure, ... Charney, D. S. (1997). Magnetic resonance imaging-based measurement of hippocampal volume in posttraumatic stress disorder related to childhood physical and sexual abuse – A preliminary report. *Biological Psychiatry, 41,* 23–32.

Bremner, J. D., Vythilingam, M., Vermetten, E., Southwick, S. M., McGlashan, T., Nazeer, A., ... Charney, D. S. (2003). MRI and PET study of deficits in hippocampal structure and function in women with childhood sexual abuse and posttraumatic stress disorder. *American Journal of Psychiatry 160,* 924–932.

Breslau, N. (2001). Outcomes of posttraumatic stress disorder. *Journal of Clinical Psychiatry, 62*(Suppl. 17), 55–59.

Brewin, C. R. (2001). A cognitive neuroscience account of posttraumatic stress disorder and its treatment. *Behaviour Research and Therapy, 39,* 373–393.

Brewin, C. R., Andrews, B., & Valentine, J. D. (2000). Meta-analysis of risk factors for posttraumatic stress disorder in trauma-exposed adults. *Journal of Consulting and Clinical Psychology, 68,* 748–766.

Brewin, C. R., Dalgleish, T., & Joseph, S. (1996). A dual representation theory of posttraumatic stress disorder. *Psychological Review, 103,* 670–686.

Buchanan, T. W. & Lovallo, W. R. (2001). Enhanced memory for emotional material following stress-level cortisol treatment in humans. *Psychoneuroendocrinology, 26,* 307–317.

Byrne, C. A., & Riggs, D. S. (1996). The cycle of trauma; relationship aggression in male Vietnam veterans with symptoms of posttraumatic stress disorder. *Violence and Victims, 11,* 213–225.

Cahill, L., Babinsky, R., Markowitsch, H. J., & McGaugh, J. L. (1995). The amygdala and emotional memory. *Nature, 377,* 295–296.

Cahill, L., Prins, B., Weber, M., & McGaugh, J. L. (1994). Beta-adrenergic activation and memory for emotional events. *Nature, 371,* 702–704.

Cardinal, R. N., Parkinson, J. A., Hall, J., Everitt, B. J. (2002). Emotion and motivation: The role of the amygdala, ventral striatum, and prefrontal cortex. *Neuroscience & Biobehavioral Reviews, 26,* 321–352.

Castles, S., & Miller, M. J. (1993). *The age of migration: International population movements in the modern world.* New York, NY: Guilford Press.

Catani, C., Gerwirtz, A. H,, Wieling, E., Schauer, E., Elbert ,T., & Neuner, F. (2010). Tsunami, war, and cumulative risk in the life of Sri Lankan school children. *Child Development, 81,* 1176–1191.

Catani, C., Schauer, E., Elbert, T., Missmahl, I., Bette, J. P., Neuner, F. (2009). War trauma, child labor, and family violence: Life adversities and PTSD in a sample of school children in Kabul. *Journal of Traumatic Stress, 22,* 163–171.

Cienfuegos, J., & Monelli, C. (1983). The testimony of political repression as a therapeutic instrument. *American Journal of Orthopsychiatry, 53,* 43–51.

Conway, M. A. (2001). Sensory-perceptual episodic memory and its context: autobiographical memory. *Philosophical Transactions of the Royal Society of London Series B: Biological Science, 356,* 1375–1384.

Conway, M. A., & Pleydell-Pearce, C. W. (2000). The construction of autobiographical memories in the self-memory system. *Psychological Review, 107,* 261–288.

Courtois, C. A., Ford, J. D. (2009). *Treating complex traumatic stress disorders: An evidence-based guide.* New York, NY: Guilford Press.

Cunningham, M., & Cunningham, J. D. (1997). Patterns of symptomatology and patterns of torture and trauma experiences in resettled refugees. *Australian and New Zealand Journal of Psychiatry, 31,* 555–565.

Darwin, C. (1998). *The expression of the emotions in man and animals.* New York, NY: Oxford University Press (Original work published 1872).

David Mendel. Polymathic cardiologist. (2007, March 20). *The Independent.* Retrieved from http://www.independent.co.uk

De Bellis, M. (2002). Developmental traumatology: a contributory mechanism for alcohol and substance use disorders. *Psychoneuroendocrinology, 27,* 155–170.

De Bellis, M. D., Baum, A. S., Birmaher, B., Keshavan, M. S., Eccard, C. H., Boring, A. M., ... Ryan, N. D. (1999). AE Bennett Research Award. Developmental traumatology. Part I: Biological stress systems. *Biological Psychiatry, 15,* 1259–1270.

Deblinger, E., Steer, R. A., & Lippmann, J. (1999). Two-year follow-up study of cognitive and behavioural therapy for sexually abused children suffering post-traumatic stress symptoms. *Child Abuse & Neglect, 23,* 1271–1378.

de Quervain, D. J.-F., Henke, K. Aerni, A., Treyer, V., McGaugh, J. L., Berthold, T., ... Hock, C. (2003). Glucocorticoid-induced impairment of declarative memory retrieval is associated with reduced blood flow in the medial temporal lobe. *European Journal of Neuroscience, 17,* 1296–1302.

de Quervain, D. J.-F., Roozendaal, B., & McGaugh, J. L. (1998). Stress and glucocorticoids impair retrieval of long-term spatial memory. *Nature, 394,* 787–790.

de Quervain, D. J.-F., Roozendaal, B., Nitsch, R. M., McGaugh, J. L., & Hock, C. (2000). Acute cortisone administration impairs retrieval of long-term declarative memory in humans. *Nature Neuroscience, 3,* 313–314.

Derriennic, J. P. (1971). Theory and ideologies of violence. *Journal of Peace Research, 8,* 361–374.

De Waal, A (1988). The sanity factor: Expatriate behavior on African relief programs. *Refugee Participation Network,* Network Paper 2b, 1 RSC/QEH.

Dube, S .R., Felitti, V. J., Chapman, D. P., Giles, W. H., & Anda, R. F. (2003). Childhood abuse, neglect and household dysfunction and the risk of illicit drug use: the Adverse Childhood Experience Study. *Pediatrics, 111,* 564–572.

Dunmore, E., Clark, D. M., & Ehlers, A. (2001). A prospective examination of the role of cognitive factors in persistent posttraumatic stress disorder (PTSD) after physical or sexual assault. *Behaviour Research and Therapy, 39,* 1063–1084.

Dutra, L., Bureau, J.-F., Holmes, B., Lyubchik, A., & Lyons-Ruth, K. (2009). Quality of early care and childhood trauma: A prospective study of developmental pathways to dissociation. *Journal of Nervous and Mental Disease, 197,* 383–390.

Dyregrov, A., Gupta, L., Gjestad, R., & Mukanoheli, E. (2000). Trauma exposure and psychological reactions to genocide among Rwandan children. *Journal of Traumatic Stress, 13,* 3–21.

Eckart, C., Stoppel, C., Kaufmann, J., Tempelmann, C., Hinrichs, H., Elbert, T., ... Kolassa, I. T. (2010). Structural alterations in lateral prefrontal, parietal and posterior midline regions of men with chronic posttraumatic stress disorder. *Journal of Psychiatry and Neuroscience, 35,* 10010–10020.

Egeland, B. (2009). Taking stock: childhood emotional maltreatment and developmental psychopathology. *Child Abuse & Neglect, 33,* 22–26.

Ehlers, A., & Clark, D. M. (2000). A cognitive model of posttraumatic stress disorder. *Behaviour Research and Therapy, 38,* 319–345.

Elbert, T., & Rockstroh, B. (2003). Stress factors: The science of our flexible responses to an unpredictable world. *Nature, 421,* 477–478.

Elbert, T., & Schauer, M. (2002). Burnt into memory. *Nature, 412,* 883.

Elbert, T., Schauer, M., Schauer, E., Huschka, B., Hirth, M., & Neuner, F. (2009). Trauma-related impairment in children – An epidemiological survey in Sri Lankan provinces affected by two decades of civil war and unrest. *Child Abuse & Neglect, 33,* 238–246.

Elbert, T., Weierstall, R., & Schauer, M. (2010). Fascination violence – on mind and brain of man hunters. *European Archives of Psychiatry and Clinical Neuroscience, 260,* 100–105.

Ertl, V., Pfeiffer, A., Saile, R., Schauer, E., Elbert, T., Neuner, F. (2010). Validation of a mental health assessment in an African conflict population. *Psychological Assessment, 22,* 318–324.

Ertl, V., Pfeiffer, A., Schauer, E., Elbert, T., Neuner, F. (2011). The challenge of living on: Psychopathology and its mediating influence on the readjustment of former child soldiers. Manuscript submitted for publication.

Farley, M., & Keaney J. C. (1997). Physical symptoms, somatization, and dissociation in women survivors of childhood sexual assault. *Women Health, 25,* 33–45.

Foa, E. B. (1995). *Post-Traumatic Stress Diagnostic Scale (PDS).* Minneapolis, MN: National Computer Systems.

Foa, E. B., Dancu, C. V., Hembree, E. A., Jaycox, L. H., Meadows, E. A., & Street, G. P. (1999). A comparison of exposure therapy, stress inoculation training, and their combination for reducing posttraumatic stress disorder in female assault victims. *Journal of Consulting and Clinical Psychology, 67,* 194–200.

Foa, E. B., Davidson, J. R. T., & Frances, A. (1999). The expert consensus guideline series. Treatment of Posttraumatic Stress disorder. *Journal of Clinical Psychiatry, 60,* 4–76.

Foa, E. B., Hearst-Ikeda, D., & Perry, K. J. (1995). Evaluation of a brief cognitive-behavioral program for the prevention of chronic PTSD in recent assault victims. *Journal of Consulting and Clinical Psychology, 63,* 948–955.

Foa, E. B., & Kozak, M. J. (1986). Emotional processing of fear: Exposure to corrective information. *Psychological Bulletin, 99,* 20–35.

Foa, E. B., Molnar, C., & Cashman, L. (1995). Change in rape narratives during exposure therapy for posttraumatic stress disorder. *Journal of Traumatic Stress, 4,* 675–690.

Foa, E. B., Riggs, D. S., & Gershuny, B. S. (1995). Arousal, numbing, and intrusion: symptom structure of PTSD following assault. *American Journal of Psychiatry, 152,* 116–120.

Foa, E. B., & Rothbaum, B. O. (1998). *Treating the trauma of rape: Cognitive-behavioral therapy for PTSD.* New York, NY: Guilford Press.

Foa, E. B., Rothbaum, B. O., Riggs, D. S., & Murdock, T. B. (1991). Treatment of posttraumatic stress disorder in rape victims: A comparison between cognitive-behavioral procedures and counseling. *Journal of Consulting and Clinical Psychology, 59,* 715–723.

Forbes Martin, S. (1991). *Refugee women.* London & New Jersey: Zed Books.

Frankl, V. (1946). *Ein Psycholog erlebt das Konzentrationslager* [A psychologist's experience of a concentration camp]. Vienna: Verlag für Jugend und Volk.

Friedman, M. J. (2000). *Posttraumatic stress disorder – The latest assessment and treatment strategies.* Compact Clinicals. New York, NY: APA.

Friedman, M. J. (2010). PTSD revisions proposed for DSM-5, with input from array of experts. *Psychiatric News, 45,* 8.

Garcia-Peltoniemi, R. E. (1991). Clinical manifestations of psychopathology. In *Mental health services for refugees.* Rockville, MD: US Department of Health and Human Services, National Institute of Mental Health.

Gilbert, P., & Procter, S. (2006). Compassionate mind training for people with high shame and self-criticism: Overview and pilot study of a group therapy approach. *Clinical Psychology & Psychotherapy, 13,* 353–379.

Gola, H., Engler, H., Schauer, M., Adenauer, H., Elbert, T., Kolassa, I. T. (in press). Victims of rape show increased cortisol responses to trauma reminders: A study in individuals with war- and torture-related PTSD. *Psychneuroendocrinology.*

Hariri AR, Bookheimer SY, Mazziotta JC. (2000). Modulating emotional response: Effects of a neocortical network on the limbic system. *Neuroreport, 11,* 43–48.

Harrell-Bond, B. E. (1986). *Imposing aid: Emergency assistance to refugees.* Oxford: Oxford University Press.

Harrell-Bond, B (2002). Can humanitarian work with refugees be humane? *Human Rights Quarterly, 24,* 51–85.

Harvey, A. G., & Bryant, R. A. (1999). A qualitative investigation of the organization of traumatic memories. *British Journal of Clinical Psychology, 38,* 401–405.

Hensel-Dittman, D., Schauer, M., Ruf, M., Catani, C., Odenwald, M., Elbert, T., Neuner, F. (in press). The treatment of traumatized victims of war and torture: A randomized controlled comparison of Narrative Exposure Therapy and Stress Inoculation Training. *Psychotherapy and Psychosomatics.*

Herman, J. L. (1992a). Complex PTSD: A syndrome in survivors of prolonged and repeated trauma. *Journal of Traumatic Stress, 5,* 377–391.

Herman, J. L. (1992b). *Trauma and recovery.* New York, NY: Basic Books.

Holmes, J. (1999). Defensive and creative uses of narrative in psychotherapy: An attachment perspective. In G. Roberts (Ed.), *Healing stories: Narrative in psychiatry and psychotherapy* (pp. 49–66). Oxford: Oxford University Press.

Howe, M. L., Courage, M. L., & Peterson, C. (1994). How can I remember when "I" wasn't there: Long-term retention of traumatic experiences and emerge of the cognitive self. *Consciousness and Cognition, 3,* 327–355.

Jaffee, S. R. (2005). Family violence and parent psychopathology. Implications for children's socioemotional development and resilience. In S. Goldstein, R. B. Brooks (Eds.), *Handbook of resilience in children* (pp. 149–163). New York, NY: Springer.

Jaycox, L. H., Foa, E. B., & Morral, A. R. (1998). Influence of emotional engagement and habituation on exposure therapy for PTSD. *Journal of Consulting and Clinical Psychology, 66,* 185–192.

Jones, D. P. H., & Krugman, R. D. (1986). Can a three-year-old child bear witness to her sexual assault and attempted murder? *Child Abuse & Neglect, 10,* 253–258.

Kaminer, D. (2006). Healing processes in trauma narratives: a review. *South African Journal of Psychology, 36*(3), 481–499.

Karunakara, U., Neuner, F., Schauer, M., Singh, K., Hill, K., Elbert, T., & Burnham, G. (2004). Traumatic events and symptoms of post-traumatic stress disorder amongst Sudanese nationals, refugees and Ugandan nationals in the West Nile. *African Health Sciences, 4,* 83–93.

Keane, T. M., Zimering, R. T., & Caddell, J. M. (1985). A behavioural formulation of posttraumatic stress disorder in combat veterans. *Behaviour Therapist, 8,* 9–12.

Kessler, R. C., Sonnega, A., Bromet, E., Hughes, M., & Nelson, C. B. (1995). Posttraumatic stress disorder in the National Comorbidity Survey. *Archives of General Psychiatry, 52,* 1048–1060.

Kiecolt-Glaser, J. K., Preacher, K. J., MacCallum, R. C., Atkinson, C., Malarkey, W. B., & Glaser, R. (2003). Chronic stress and age-related increases in the proinflammatory cytokine IL-6. *Proceedings of the National Academy of Sciences USA, 100,* 9090–9095.

Kim, J. J., & Yoon, K. S. (1998). Stress: Metaplastic effects in the hippocampus. *Trends in Neuroscience, 21,* 505–509.

Kinzie, J. D., Sack, W. H., Angell R. H., & Clarke, G. (1989). A three-year follow-up of Cambodian young people traumatized as children. *Journal of the American Academy of Child and Adolescent Psychiatry, 28,* 501–504.

Kinzl, J. F., Traweger, C., & Biebl, W. (1995). Family background and sexual abuse associated with somatization. *Psychotherapy and Psychosomatics, 64,* 82–87.

Klonsky, E. D., Oltmanns, T. F., & Turkheimer E. (2003). Deliberate self-harm in a nonclinical population: prevalence and psychological correlates. *American Journal of Psychiatry 160,* 1501–1508.

Kolassa, I. T., & Elbert, T. (2007). Structural and functional neuroplasticity in relation to traumatic stress. *Current Directions in Psychological Science, 16,* 326–329.

Kolassa I. T., Ertl, V., Kolassa, S., Onyut, L. P., & Elbert, T. (2010). Spontaneous remission from PTSD depends on the number of traumatic event types experienced. *Psychological Trauma: Theory, Research, Practice, and Policy, 2,* 169–174.

Kolassa, I. T., Wienbruch, C., Neuner, F., Schauer, M., Ruf, M., Odenwald, M., & Elbert, T. (2007). Altered oscillatory brain dynamics after repeated traumatic stress. *BMC Psychiatry, 7:*56.

Koss, M. P., Tromp, S., & Tharan, M. (1995) Traumatic memories: Empirical foundation, clinical and forensic implications. *Clinical Psychology: Research and Practice, 2, 11,* 1–132.

Krusemark, E. A., & Li, W. (2011). Do all threats work the same way? Divergent effects of fear and disgust on sensory perception and attention. *The Journal of Neuroscience, 31,* 3429–3434.

Kubany, E. S. (1994). A cognitive model of guilt typology in combat-related PTSD. *Journal of Traumatic Stress, 7,* 3–19.

Lang, P. J. (1977). Imagery in therapy: An information processing analysis of fear. *Behavior Therapy, 8,* 862–866.

Lang, P. J. (1979). A bio-informational theory of emotional imagery. *Psychophysiology, 16,* 195–512.

Lang, P. J. (1984). Dead Souls: Or why the neurobehavioral science of emotion should pay attention to cognitive science. In Th. Elbert, B. Rockstroh, W. Lutzenberger, & N. Birbaumer (Eds.), *Self-regulation of the brain and behaviour* (pp. 255–272). Berlin: Springer Verlag.

Lang, P. J. (1993). The network model of emotion: Motivational connections. In R. Wyer & T. Scrull (Eds.), *Advances in social cognition, VI.* Hillsdale, NJ: Lawrence Erlbaum Associate.

Lang, P. J., Davis, M., & Ohman, A. (2000). Fear and anxiety: Animal models and human cognitive psychophysiology. *Journal of Affective Disorders, 61,* 137–159.

LeDoux, J. E. (2000). Emotion Circuits in the brain. *Annual Review of Neuroscience, 23,* 155–184.

Levi, Primo. (1963). La tregua [the reawakening]. Torino: Einaudi.

Lieb, K., Zanarini, M., Linehan, M. M., Bohus, M. (2004). Borderline personality disorder. *The Lancet, 364,* 453–461.

Lieberman M. D., Eisenberger, N. I., Crockett, M. J., Tom, S. M., Pfeifer, J. H., Way, B. M. (2007). Putting feelings into words: affect labeling disrupts amygdala activity to affective stimuli. *Psychological Science, 18,* 421–428.

Lieberman, M. D., Hariri, A., Jarcho, J. M., Eisenberger, N. I., Bookheimer, S. Y. (2005). An fMRI investigation of race-related amygdala activity in African-American and Caucasian-American individuals. *Nature Neuroscience, 8,* 720–722.

Macdonald, G., & Leary, M. R. (2005). Why does social exclusion hurt? The relationship between social and physical pain. *Psychological Bulletin, 131,* 202–223.

Madigan, S., Bakermans-Kranenburg, M., van IJzendoorn, M., Moran, G., Pederson, D., & Benoit, D. (2006). Unresolved states of mind, anomalous parental behavior, and disorganized attachment: A review and metaanalysis of a transmission gap. *Attachment and Human Development, 8,* 89–111.

Malkki, L. H. (1995). *Purity and exile: Violence memory, and national cosmology among Hutu refugees in Tanzania.* Chicago, IL: The University of Chicago Press.

Margolin, G., & Gordis, E. B., (2000). The effects of family and community violence on children, *Annual Review of Psychology, 51,* 445–479.

Matz, K., Junghöfer, M., Elbert, T., Weber, K., Wienbruch, C., & Rockstroh, B. (2010). Adverse experiences in childhood influence brain responses to emotional stimuli in adult psychiatric patients. *International Journal of Psychophysiology, 75,* 277–286.

McClelland, J. L., McNaughton, B. L., & O'Reilly, R. C. (1995). Why there are complementary learning systems in the hippocampus and neocortex: Insights from the successes and failures of connectionist models of learning and memory. *Psychological Review, 102,* 419–457.

McEwen, B. S. (1999). Stress and hippocampal plasticity. *Annual Review of Neuroscience, 22,* 105–122.

McEwen, B. S. (2002). The end of stress as we know it. Washington, DC: Joseph Henry Press/Dana Press.

McFarlane, A. C., Atchison, M., Rafalowicz, E., & Papay, P. (1994). Physical symptoms in post-traumatic stress disorder. *Journal of Psychosomatic Research, 38,* 715–726.

McGaugh, J. L. (2002). Memory consolidation and the amygdala: A systems perspective. *Trends in Neuroscience, 25,* 456.

McLean, L. M., & Gallop, R. (2003). Implications of childhood sexual abuse for adult borderline personality disorder and complex posttraumatic stress disorder. *American Journal of Psychiatry, 160, 2,* 369–371.

McLeer, S. V., Callaghan, M., Henry, D., & Wallen, J., (1994). Psychiatric disorders in sexually abused children. *Journal of the American Academy of Child & Adolescent Psychiatry, 33,* 313–319.

McLeer, S. V., Dixon, J. F., Henry, D., Ruggiero, K., Escovitz, K., Niedda, T., & Scholle, R. (1998). Psychopathology in non-clinically referred sexually abused children. *Journal of the American Academy of Child & Adolescent Psychiatry, 37,* 1326–1333.

Meaney, M. (2008). Maternal care and hippocampal plasticity: Evidence for experience-dependent structural plasticity, altered synaptic functioning, and differential responsiveness to glucocorticoids and stress. *Journal of Neuroscience, 28*(23), 6037–6045.

Meaney, M., Aitken, D., van Berkel, C., Bhatnagar, C., & Sapolsky, R. (1988). Effects of neonatal handling on age-related impairments associated with the hippocampus. *Science, 239,* 766–770.

Metcalfe, J., & Jacobs, W. (1996). A hot-system/cool-system view of memory under stress. *PTSD Research Quarterly, 7,* 1–3.

Mills, R. S. L. (2005). Taking stock of the developmental literature on shame. *Developmental Review, 25,* 26–63.

Misch, P., Phillips, M., Evans, P., & Berelowitz, M. (1993). Trauma in pre-school children: A clinical account. In G. Forrest (Ed.), *Trauma and crisis management.* London: ACPP Publications.

Morrison, J. (1989) Childhood sexual histories of women with somatization disorder. *American Journal of Psychiatry, 146,* 239–241.

Nader, K., Schafe, G. E., & LeDoux, J. E. (2000). Fear memories require protein synthesis in the amygdala for consolidation after retrieval. *Nature, 406,* 722.

Neuner, F., & Elbert, T. (2007). The mental health disaster in conflict settings: Can scientific research help? *BMC Public Health, 7,* 275.

Neuner, F., Kurreck, S., Ruf, M., Odenwald, M., Elbert, T., & Schauer, M. (2009). Can asylum seekers with posttraumatic stress disorder be successfully treated? A randomized controlled pilot study, *Cognitive Behaviour Therapy, 39,* 81–91.

Neuner, F., Onyut, P. L., Ertl, V., Odenwald, M., Schauer, E., & Elbert, T. (2008). Treatment of posttraumatic stress disorder by trained lay counselors in an African refugee settlement: A randomized controlled trial. *Journal of Consulting and Clinical Psychology, 76,* 686–694.

Neuner, F,. Schauer, E., Catani, C., Ruf, M., & Elbert, T. (2006). Post-Tsunami stress: A study of posttraumatic stress disorder in children living in three severely affected regions in Sri Lanka. *Journal of Traumatic Stress, 19*, 339–347.

Neuner, F., Schauer, M., Elbert, T., & Roth, W. T. (2002). A narrative exposure treatment as intervention in a Macedonia's refugee camp: a case report. *Journal of Behavioural and Cognitive Psychotherapy, 30*, 205–209.

Neuner, F., Schauer, M., Karunakara, U., Klaschik, C., Robert C., & Elbert, T. (2004a) Psychological trauma and evidence for enhanced vulnerability for PTSD through previous trauma in West Nile refugees. *BMC Psychiatry, 4*, 34.

Neuner, F., Schauer, M., Klaschik, C., Karunakara, U., & Elbert, T. (2004b). A comparison of narrative exposure therapy, supportive counseling and psychoeducation for treating posttraumatic stress disorder in an African refugee settlement. *Journal of Consulting and Clinical Psychology, 72*, 579–587.

Nutt, D. J., & Malizia, A. L. (2004). Structural and functional brain changes in posttraumatic stress disorder. *Journal of Clinical Psychiatry, 65*(Suppl. 1), 11–17.

Onyut, P. L., Neuner, F., Ertl, V., Schauer, E., Odenwald, M., & Elbert, T. (2009). Trauma, poverty and mental health among Somali and Rwandese refugees living in an African refugee settlement – an epidemiological study. *Conflict and Health, 3*, 6.

Onyut, L. P., Neuner, F., Schauer, E., Ertl, V., Odenwald, M., Schauer, M., & Elbert, T. (2004). The Nakivale Camp Mental Health Project: Building local competency for psychological assistance to traumatised refugees. *Intervention, 2*(2), 90–107.

Onyut, P. L., Neuner, F., Schauer, E., Ertl, V., Odenwald, M., Schauer, M., & Elbert, T. (2005). Narrative Exposure Therapy as a treatment for child war survivors with posttraumatic stress disorder: Two case reports and a pilot study in an African refugee settlement. *BMC Psychiatry, 5*, 7.

Ozer, E. J., Best, S. R., Lipsey, T. L., & Weiss, D. S. (2003). Predictors of posttraumatic stress disorder and symptoms in adults: A meta-analysis. *Psychological Bulletin, 129*, 52–73.

Panksepp, J. (2003). Neuroscience: Feeling the pain of social loss. *Science, 302(5643)*, 237–239.

Papageorgiou, V., Frangou-Garunovic, A., Iordanidou, R., Yule, W., Smith, P., & Vostanis P. (2000). War trauma and psychopathology in Bosnian refugee children. *European Child and Adolescent Psychiatry, 9*, 84–90.

Pavlov, I. P. (1927). *Conditioned Reflexes: An Investigation of the Physiological Activity of the Cerebral Cortex.* Transl. and ed. by G. V. Anrep. London, UK: Oxford University Press.

Pelcovitz, D., van der Kolk, B., Roth, S., Mandel, F., Kaplan, S., & Resick, P. (1997). Development of a criteria set and a structured interview for disorders of extreme stress (SIDES). *Journal of Traumatic Stress, 10*, 3–16.

Pennebaker, J. W., & Seagal, J. D. (1999). Forming a story: The health benefits of narrative. *Journal of Clinical Psychology, 55*, 1243–1254.

Peterson, C. (1996). The preschool child witness: Errors in account of traumatic injury. *Canadian Journal of Behavioural Science, 28*, 36–42.

Pynoos, R. S., & Nader, K., (1989). Children's memory and proximity to violence. *Journal of the American Academy of Child & Adolescent Psychiatry, 28*, 236–241.

Reviere, S. L. (1996). *Memory of childhood trauma: A clinician's guide to the literature.* New York, NY: Guilford Press.

Riggs, D. S., Byrne, C. A., Weathers, F. W., & Litz, B. T. (1998). The quality of the intimate relationships of male Vietnam veterans: Problems associated with posttraumatic stress disorder. *Journal of Traumatic Stress, 11*, 87–101.

Robinaugh, D. J., & McNally, R. J. (2010). Autobiographical memory for shame or guilt provoking events: association with psychological symptoms. *Behaviour Research and Therapy, 48*, 646–652.

Robinson, J. A. (1992). First experience memories: Contexts and function in personal histories. In M. A. Conway, D. C. Rubin, H. Spinnler, & W. A. Wagenaar (Eds.), *Theoretical perspectives on autobiographical memories* (pp. 223–239). Dodrecht, The Netherlands: Kluwer Academics.

Robjant, K., & Fazel, M. (2010). The emerging evidence for Narrative Exposure Therapy: A review. *Clinical Psychology Reviews, 30*, 1030–1039.

Roozendaal, B., de Quervain, D. J.-F., Ferry, B., Setlow, B., McGaugh, J. L. (2001). Basolateral amygdala-nucleus accumbens interactions in mediating glucocorticoid enhancement of memory consolidation. *Journal of Neuroscience, 21*, 2518–2525.

Roozendaal, B., Griffith, Q. K., Buranday, J., de Quervain, D. J.-F., & McGaugh, J. L. (2003). The hippocampus mediates glucocorticoid-induced retrieval impairments of spatial memory: Dependence on the basolateral amygdala. *Proceedings of the National Academy of Science of the U S A, 100*, 1328–1333.

Rosenthal, G. (1997). Traumatische Familienvergangenheiten [Traumatic family backgrounds]. In G. Rosenthal (Ed.), *Der Holocaust im Leben von drei Generationen [The Holocaust in the lives of three generations].* Gießen, Germany: Psychosozial-Verlag.

Rothbaum B. O., Foa, E. B., Rigge, D. S., Murdoch, T., & Walsh, W. A. (1992). Prospective examination of post-traumatic stress disorder in rape victims. *Journal of Traumatic Stress, 5*, 455–475.

Rothbaum, B. O., & Foa, B. F. (1999). Exposure therapy for PTSD. *PTSD Research Quarterly, 10*(2), 1–3.

Rudy, J. W., & Sutherland, R. J. (1994). The memory coherence problem, configural associations, and the hippocampal system. In D. L. Schachter & E. Tulving (Eds.). *Memory systems* (pp. 119–146). Cambridge, MA: MIT Press.

Ruf, M., Schauer, M., & Elbert, T. (2009). Raum für den Dritten – Sprachmittler in der Therapie von Flüchtlingen. In *Psychotherapie zu Dritt, Zeitschrift für Flüchtlingspolitik 4*, Sonderheft 125, 10–14.

Ruf, M., Schauer, M., Neuner, F., Catani, C., Schauer, E., & Elbert, T. (2010). Narrative Exposure Therapy for 7- to 16-year-olds – a randomized controlled trial with traumatized refugee children. *Journal of Traumatic Stress, 23*, 437–445.

Saigh, P. A. (1991). The development of post-traumatic stress disorder following four different types of traumatizations. *Behaviour Research & Therapy, 29*, 213–216.

Saigh, P. A. (1992). The behavioural treatment of child and adolescent post-traumatic stress disorder. *Advances in Behaviour Research & Therapy, 14*, 247–275.

Saigh, P. A., Yule, W., & Inamdar, S. C. (1996). Imaginal flooding of traumatized children and adolescents. *Journal of School Psychology, 34*, 163–183.

Sapolsky, R. M. (1999). Glucocorticoids, stress, and their adverse neurological effects: Relevance to aging. *Experimental Gerontology, 34*(6), 721–732.

Schaaf, K .K., & McCanne, T. R. (1994). Childhood abuse, body image disturbance, and eating disorders. *Child Abuse & Neglect, 18,* 607–615.

Schaal, S., & Elbert, T. (2006). Ten years after the genocide: Trauma confrontation and posttraumatic stress in Rwandan adolescents. *Journal of Traumatic Stress, 19,* 95–105.

Schaal, S., Elbert, T., & Neuner, F. (2009). Narrative Exposure Therapy versus group Interpersonal Psychotherapy: A controlled clinical trial with orphaned survivors of the Rwandan genocide. *Psychotherapy and Psychosomatics, 78,* 298–306.

Schacter, D. L. (1996). Searching for memory: The brain, the mind and the past. New York, NY: Basic Books.

Schalinski, I., Elbert ,T., Schauer, M. (2011). Female dissociative responding to extreme sexual violence in a chronic crisis setting: The case of Eastern Congo. *Journal of Traumatic Stress, 24,* 235–238. doi: 10.1002/jts.20631

Schauer, E., Neuner, F., Elbert, T., Ertl, V., Onyut, L., Odenwald, M., & Schauer, M. (2004). Narrative exposure therapy in children – A case study. *Intervention, 2*(1), 18–32.

Schauer, M., & Elbert, T. (2010). Dissociation following traumatic stress: Etiology and treatment. *Zeitschrift für Psychologie/ Journal of Psychology, 218,* 109–127.

Schauer, M., Elbert, T., Gotthardt, S., Rockstroh, B., Odenwald, M., Neuner, F. (2006). Wiedererfahrung durch Psychotherapie modifiziert Geist und Gehirn. *Verhaltenstherapie, 16,* 96–103.

Schauer, M., Elbert, T., Neuner, F. (2007). Interaktion von Neurowissenschaftlichen Erkenntnissen und Psychotherapeutischen Einsichten am Beispiel von Angst und traumatischem Stress. In R. Becker, H.-P. Wunderlich (Eds.), *Wie wirkt Psychotherapie: Forschungsgrundlagen für die Praxis* (pp. 87–108). Stuttgart/ New York: Thieme-Verlag.

Schauer, M., Neuner, F., Karunakara, U., Klaschik, C., Robert, C., & Elbert, T. (2003). PTSD and the "building block" effect of psychological trauma among West Nile Africans. *ESTSS (European Society for Traumatic Stress Studies) Bulletin, 10* (2), 5–6.

Schauer, M., Schauer, E. (2010). Trauma-focused public mental-health interventions: A paradigm shift in humanitarian assistance and aid work. In E. Martz (Ed), *Trauma rehabilitation after war and conflict* (pp. 361–430). New York, NY: Springer.

Segerstrom, S. C., & Miller, G. E. (2004). Psychological stress and the human immune system: A meta-analytic study of 30 years of inquiry. *Psychological Bulletin, 130,* 601–630.

Shin, L. M., Rauch, S. L., & Pitman, R. K. (2006). Amygdala, medial prefrontal cortex, and hippocampal function in PTSD. *Annals of the New York Academy of Sciences, 1071,* 67–79.

Shum, M. S. (1998). The role of temporal landmarks in autobiographical memory processes. *Psychological Bulletin, 124,* 423–442.

Smolak, L,, & Murnen, S. K. (2002). A meta-analytic examination of the relationship between child sexual abuse and eating disorders. *International Journal of Eating Disorders, 31,* 136–150.

Somasundaram, D. J. (1993). *Child trauma.* Jaffna: University of Jaffna, Sri Lanka.

Sommershof, A., Aichinger, H., Engler, E,. Adenauer ,H., Catani, C., Boneberg, E. M., ... Kolassa, I. (2009). Lack of naive and regulatory T cells in posttraumatic stress disorder patients. *Brain, Behavior, and Immunity, 23,* 117–1123.

Squire, L. R. (1994). Declarative and nondeclarative memory: Multiple brain systems supporting learning and memory. In D. L. Schacter & E. Tulving (Eds.), *Memory Systems* (pp. 207–228). Cambridge, MA: MIT Press.

Staub, E. (1998). Breaking the cycle of genocidal violence: Healing and reconciliation, In J. H. Harvey (Ed.), *Perspectives on loss: A source book: Death, dying, and bereavement.* Philadelphia, PA: Brunner/Mazel, Inc.

Steil, R. (2000). Post-traumatische Belastungsstörung [Posttraumatic stress disorder]. In M. Hatzinger (Ed.), *Kognitive Verhaltenstherapie psychischer Störungen* [Cognitive behavior therapy of psychological disorders]. Weinheim, Germany: PVU.

Stein, A. (1993). *Hidden children.* London: Viking.

Streans, S. D. (1992). *Psychological distress and relief work: who helps the helpers?* Oxford: Refugees Studies Programme, University of Oxford.

Stuewig, J., & McCloskey, L. A. (2005). The relation of child maltreatment to shame and guilt among adolescents: psychological routes to depression and delinquency. *Child Maltreatment, 10,* 324–336.

Sullivan, M. A., Saylor, C. F., & Foster, K. Y. (1991). Post-hurricane adjustment of preschoolers and their families. *Advances in Behaviour Research and Therapy, 13,* 163–171.

Summerfield, D. (1997). Legacy of war: Beyond "trauma" to the social fabric. *The Lancet, 349,* 1568.

Summerfield, D. (2004). Cross cultural perspectives on the medicalitsation of human suffering. In G. Rosen (Ed.), *Posttraumatic stress disorder. Issues and controversies.* New York, NY: John Wiley.

Tandon, Y. (1984). Ugandan refugees in Kenya: A community of enforced self-reliance. *Disasters, 8,* 267–271.

Tangney, J. P., Stuewig, J., & Mashek, D. J. (2007). Moral emotions and moral behavior. *Annual Review of Psychology, 58,* 345–372.

Tauber, C. D. (2003). *Psychological trauma, physical health and conflict resolution in Croatia, Serbia and Bosnia: Lessons for the future.* Retrieved on 17.02.2003 from http://www.conflic-tres. org/vol 184/tauber.htm

Teicher, M. H., Andersen, S. L., Polcari, A., Anderson, C. M., & Navalta, C. P. (2002). Developmental neurobiology of childhood stress and trauma. *Psychiatric Clinics of North America, 25,* 397–326.

Terr, L. (1993). *Unchained memories.* New York, NY: Basic Books.

Terr, L. C. (1988). What happens to early memories of trauma? A study of twenty children under age five at the time of documented traumatic events. *Journal of the American Academy of Child and Adolescent Psychiatry, 27,* 96–104.

Tessler, M., & Nelson, K. (1994). Making memories: The influence of joint encoding on later recall by young children. *Consciousness and Cognition, 3,* 307–326.

Thabet, A. A., & Vostanis, P. (1999). Post-traumatic stress reactions in children of war. *The Journal of Child Psychology and Psychiatry, 40,* 385–391.

Thabet, A. A., & Vostanis, P. (2000). Post traumatic stress disorder reactions in children of war: A longitudinal study. *Child Abuse and Neglect, 24,* 291–298.

Tulving, E. (2001). Episodic memory and common sense: how far apart? *Philosophical Transactions of the Royal Society of London Series B: Biological Science, 356,* 1505–1515.

Turner, S. (1999). *Angry young men in camps: Gender, age and class relations among Burundian refugees in Tanzania* (Working Paper No. 9). Roskilde: Roskilde University, Institute of Development Studies.

UNHCR. (2002). *Extensive abuse of West African refugee children reported.* Retrieved on June 9, 2002, from http://www.unhcr.ch/

UNICEF. (2001). *The state of the world's children 2001.* New York, NY: Author.

United Nations. (1984). *Convention against torture and other cruel, inhuman or degrading treatment or punishment.* Retrieved on January, 7, 2003, from http://www.unhchr.ch/html/menu3/b/h_cat39.htm

van der Kolk, B. A. (1994). The body keeps the score: Memory and the evolving psychobiology of posttraumatic stress. *Harvard Review of Psychiatry, 1,* 253–265.

van der Kolk, B. (1995). Dissociation and the fragmentary nature of traumatic memories: overview and exploratory study. *Journal of Traumatic Stress, 8,* 4.

van der Kolk, B. A. (1996). Trauma and memory. In B. A. van der Kolk, A. C. McFarlane, & L. Weisaeth (Eds.), *Traumatic stress.* New York, NY: Guilford Press.

van der Kolk, B. A. (1997). The psychobiology of posttraumatic stress disorder. *Journal of Clinical Psychiatry, 58*(Suppl 9), 16–24.

van der Kolk, B. A., Roth, S., Pelcovitz, D., & Mandel, F. (1993). *Complex PTSD: Results of the PTSD field trials for DSM-IV.* Washington, DC: American Psychiatric Association.

Vitanza, S., & Vogel, S. (1995). Distress and symptoms of posttraumatic stress disorder in abused women. *Violence and Victims, 10,* 23–34.

Wagenaar, W. A. & Groeneweg, J. (1990). The memory of concentration camp survivors. *Applied Cognitive Psychology, 4,* 77–87.

Waldron, S. (1987). Blaming the Refugees (PhD Thesis, Harvard University). *RSP/BRC Refugee Issues, 3,* No. 3.

Walker, E. A., Katon, W. J., Hansom, J., Harrop-Griffiths, J., Holm, L., Jones, M. L., Hickok, L., Jemelka, R. P. (1992) Medical and psychiatric symptoms in women with childhood sexual abuse. *Psychosomatic Medicine, 54,* 658–664.

Weine, S. M., Becker, D. F., McGlashan, T. H., Laub, D., Lazrove, S., & Vojvoda, D. (1995). Psychiatric consequences of "ethnic cleansing": Clinical assessments and trauma testimonies of newly resettled Bosnian refugees. *American Journal of Psychiatry, 152,* 536–542.

Weine, S. M., Kulenovic, A. D., Pavkovic, I., & Gibbons, R. (1998). Testimony psychotherapy in Bosnian refugees: A pilot study. *American Journal of Psychiatry, 155,* 1720–1726.

Weine, S., & Laub, D. (1995). Narrative constructions of historical realities in testimony with Bosnian survivors of "ethnic cleansing." *Psychiatry, 58,* 246–260.

WHO. (1993). *International classifications of diseases* (Chapter Five). Geneva: Author.

WHO. (1997). *Composite International Diagnostic Interview (CIDI).* Geneva: Author.

WHO/UNHCR. (1996). *Mental health of refugees.* Geneva: World Health Organization.]

Widom, C. S. (1999). Posttraumatic stress disorder in abused and neglected children grown up. *American Journal of Psychiatry, 156,* 1223–1229.

Widom, C. S., Czaja, S. J., & Paris, J. (2009). A prospective investigation of borderline personality disorder in abused and neglected children followed up into adulthood. *Journal of Personality Disorders, 5,* 433–446

Widom, C. S., & Morris, S. (1997). Accuracy of adult recollections of childhood victimization: Part II: Childhood sexual abuse. *Psychological Assessment, 9,* 34–46.

Widom, C. S., & Shepard, R. L. (1996). Accuracy of adult recollections of childhood victimization: Part I: Childhood physical abuse. *Psychological Assessment, 8,* 412–421.

Wiesel, E. (1996). *Interview: Holocaust survivor's storyteller.* Washington, DC: Academy of Achievement, Museum of Living History. Retrieved from http://www.achievement.org

Williams L. M. & Banyard V. L. (1999). *Trauma and memory,* Newbury Park, CA: Sage Publications.

Williams, K. D. (2007). Ostracism. *Annual Review of Psychology, 58,* 425–452.

Yehuda, R., & McFarlane, A. C. (1995). Conflict between current knowledge about posttraumatic stress disorder and its original conceptual basis. *American Journal of Psychiatry, 152,* 1705–1713.

Yule, W. (2001). Posttraumatic stress disorder in the general population and in children. *Journal of Clinical Psychiatry, 62*(Suppl. 17), 23–8.

Zlotnick, C., Rodriguez, B. F., Weisberg, R. E., Bruce, S. E., Spencer, M. A., Culpeper, L., et al. (2004). Chronicity in posttraumatic stress disorder and predictors over the course of posttraumatic stress disorder among primary care patients. *Journal of Nervous and Mental Disease, 192,* 153–159.

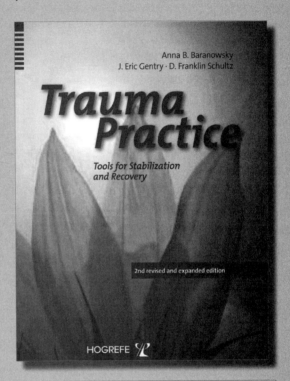
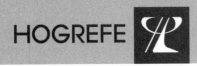